GALEN ON BLOODLETTING

GALEN ON BLOODLETTING

A study of the origins, development and validity
of his opinions, with a translation of the three works

PETER BRAIN

University of Natal

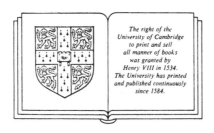

The right of the
University of Cambridge
to print and sell
all manner of books
was granted by
Henry VIII in 1534.
The University has printed
and published continuously
since 1584.

CAMBRIDGE UNIVERSITY PRESS

Cambridge

London   New York   New Rochelle
Melbourne   Sydney

CAMBRIDGE UNIVERSITY PRESS
Cambridge, New York, Melbourne, Madrid, Cape Town, Singapore, São Paulo, Delhi

Cambridge University Press
The Edinburgh Building, Cambridge CB2 8RU, UK

Published in the United States of America by Cambridge University Press, New York

www.cambridge.org
Information on this title: www.cambridge.org/9780521106542

First published 1986
This digitally printed version 2009

A catalogue record for this publication is available from the British Library

Library of Congress Cataloguing in Publication data
Brain, Peter.
Galen on bloodletting.
Partial contents: Galen's book on venesection against Erasistratus –
Galen's book on venesection against the Erasistrateans in Rome –
Galen's book on treatment by venesection.
1. Galen. 2. Bloodletting – Early works to 1800. 3. Medicine,
Greek and Roman. I. Galen. Selections. English. 1986. II. Title.
R126.G8B74 1986   615.8'99   85-25489

ISBN 978-0-521-32085-6 hardback
ISBN 978-0-521-10654-2 paperback

To J. B. B.

λέγει γάρ, Ὁ παλαιὸς χρηστότερός ἐστιν
Luke 5.39

CONTENTS

PREFACE

This work originated from an interest in the history of ideas in medicine. I wanted to find out why our forefathers, almost to a man, believed that the proper way to treat most diseases was to remove blood from the patient, and as there was to my knowledge no published translation of Galen's three bloodletting works in any modern language, I made one from the Greek of Kühn's edition, and went on to consider where his ideas came from and how they developed in the course of a long and active life. The material was used in 1978 as a dissertation for the degree of M.A. in classics from the University of Natal. Subsequently the translations have been revised, and the discussion rewritten to make it more accessible to the general reader. An introductory chapter on Galen's system of pathology, based on subsequent reading, has been added, and the passages quoted in the text in Greek and in modern languages other than English have been translated. Although unfamiliar old terms are explained when first encountered, they have all been collected into a glossary for easy reference, together with such modern technical terms as may be unfamiliar to the non-specialist.

Kühn's text is corrupt in many places, and only one of the three works has had any critical attention. I have therefore examined a number of the manuscripts and early printed editions, which clear up some of the difficulties. I must make it clear, however, that the only aim has been to improve the translations, not to establish texts; I am not a philologist, even by inclination.

I am greatly indebted to the late Dr C. R. S. Harris, Dr Theodore James, Professor G. E. R. Lloyd, Dr Vivian Nutton, the late Dr Walter Pagel, and an anonymous reader for Cambridge University Press for many suggestions. Unlike Galen's friends, however (see p. 74) they are in no way responsible for the defects of the final product. Mr Robin Price of the Wellcome Institute for the History of Medicine was most helpful on manuscripts and early editions of Galen, as were the authorities of the Vatican Library. For microfilms of manuscripts and permission to use them I thank also the Biblioteca Ambrosiana, Milan, the Biblioteca Marciana, Venice, the Biblioteca Laurenziana, Florence, and the library of the University of Bologna. Mr Abel Moses of the Natal Institute of Immunology was indefatigable in arranging inter-library loans. Professor B. X. de Wet agreed without hesitation to supervise the original somewhat outlandish project, and made many valuable suggestions for the early drafts of the translations. I thank the University of Natal for a generous grant for texts and microfilms, Mrs Joy McGill who got them for me, and my wife for her encouragement.

P.B.

Durban
April 1985

NOTE ON ABBREVIATIONS AND REFERENCES

(For abbreviations used in the section of translations only, see pp. xii–xiii)

K: *Claudii Galeni Opera Omnia, editionem curavit C. G. Kühn*, 20 vols., reprinted 1964, Hildesheim, Olms. The seventeenth and eighteenth volumes are double, and are referred to as a and b. (Facsimile of original Leipzig edition, 1821–33.)

L: *Oeuvres complètes d'Hippocrate: traduction nouvelle, avec le texte grec en regard* . . . par É. Littré. 10 vols., reprinted 1962, Amsterdam, Hakkert. (Facsimile of original Paris edition, 1839–61.)

LSJ: Liddell, H. G., Scott, R., and Jones, H. S., *A Greek–English lexicon*, 9th ed., Oxford, Clarendon Press, 1968.

OCD: *The Oxford classical dictionary*, ed. N. G. L. Hammond and H. H. Scullard, 2nd ed., Oxford, Clarendon Press, 1970.

When a book or paper is cited for the first time, the reference appears in the usual way in a footnote. If the same work is cited again, only the author's surname and the page are mentioned, with the year of publication if there is more than one work by the same author. There are thus no *op. cit.* references; a reader who wants the reference should look, not back to its first mention, but to the list of references at the end of the book, where all the works appear in alphabetical order of authors' names.

The figures in the margins of the translations, prefixed by K, indicate approximately the pagination in Kühn's eleventh volume. The numbering of sections or chapters within each translated work follows Kühn; it is not Galen's.

Individual works of Galen are often referred to, following tradition, by their Latin titles.

NOTE ON MANUSCRIPTS AND EDITIONS

(NOTE: I = De Venae Sectione adversus Erasistratum
    II = De Venae Sectione adversus Erasistrateos Romae degentes
    III = De Curandi Ratione per Venae Sectionem)

The principal manuscripts, with the exception of Athos, Iveron Mon. 4309, 189 (for III) have been examined, but no attempt has been made to study the editions exhaustively. Only a few of them have been consulted at points of difficulty with Kühn's text not cleared up by the MSS, or otherwise of interest. I follow Sider and McVaugh[1] in quoting other readings only when they give a sense appreciably different from that of Kühn's Greek. For works I and III I have revised my original translations from Kühn in the light of a collation of the MSS. R. F. Kotrc[2] has prepared a critical edition of II using the MSS A, U and M, and has supplemented this by two further publications[3] in which he refers to the MS, here called La, of which he was unaware when preparing his first study. Since his work on La has not been exhaustive, I have revised my translation of II, which was originally from Kühn, from a collation of Kotrc's (1970) text with the readings of La. The result is that I usually mention Kotrc only when disagreeing with him; since this could give a very false impression, I must acknowledge here my debt to his careful work.

MANUSCRIPTS

A   Milan, Ambrosiana graec. B 108 Sup. Contains II from K 222, line 18; I; and III from beginning to K xi, 308, line 9.
U   Vatican, Urbinas gr. 70. Contains II, I; III as A.
M   Venice, Marciana 279 (now 705). Contents as for U, except that II from K 228, line 7 to 233, line 13 is missing.
These three MSS are very closely related. Kotrc (1970) has shown that U and M both descend from A through a lost intermediary.
La Florence, Laurentiana Plut. 74, 22. Contains II from beginning to K 191, line 2; K 198, line 16 to K 229, line 8; K 236, line 3 to 244, line 15; and the whole of III.

[1] D. Sider and M. McVaugh, 'Galen on tremor, palpitation, spasm and rigor', *Trans. Stud. Coll. Phys. Philad.* n.s. 6 (1979) 183–210.
[2] R. F. Kotrc, 'Galen's On Phlebotomy against the Erasistrateans in Rome', PhD thesis, University of Washington, 1970.
[3] R. F. Kotrc, 'Critical notes on Galen's De venae sectione adversus Erasistrateos Romae degentes (K xi, 187–249)', *Class. Quart.* 23 (1973) 369–74; *idem*, 'A new fragment of Erasistratus' 'Η ΤΩΝ 'ΥΓΙΕΙΝΩΝ ΠΡΑΓΜΑΤΕΙΑ', *Rh. Mus.* 120 (1977) 159–61.

La and A represent relatively independent traditions.

Bologna, Biblioteca Universitaria 3636 has been examined; it contains a condensed paraphrase, in Greek, of III, which is not generally useful.

PRINTED EDITIONS

Ald *Galeni librorum pars quarta*, Venetiis, apud Aldum, n.d. (*c.* 1525). Greek text of the three works.

Ch *Hippocratis Coi et Claudii Galeni . . . Opera*, ed. R. Chartier, Paris, A. Pralard, 1679. Vol. x. Greek text with Latin translation.

Fu *Claudii Galeni . . . aliquot opera, a Leonharto Fuchsio Tubingensis . . . Latinate donata . . .*, Paris, 1549. Latin translation only, with an extensive commentary.

Ju *Galeni librorum sexta classis . . . septima hac nostra editione.* Venetiis, apud Iuntas, 1597. Latin translation only, with notes. For I and II the translation is by Joseph Tectander, 'denuo ab Augustino Gadaldino ad Graecorum exemplarium fidem emendatus'. III is in the version of Theodoricus Gaudanus, but differs from his earlier version in Ga.

Ga *Galeni de curandi ratione per sanguinis missionem liber, Theodorico Gaudano interprete*, Paris 1529. Latin translation.

NOTE: Accents are not written when quoting from the MSS, since it is frequently impossible to be sure of them. Although the words are separated by spaces in the quotations, in the interests of the reader, this is not done in any of the MSS.

CHAPTER 1

Galen and his system:
an introduction

Galen (c. AD 129–200) was a Greek from Pergamon in Asia Minor. Because of his habit of putting autobiographical details into his works, we know that he was the son of a prosperous architect, Nikon, who named him Galenos (mild),[1] perhaps in the hope that he would turn out different from his mother, who was a shrew. He speaks of his father with respect; he gave him an excellent education in literature, philosophy and the sciences, and finally sent him to Alexandria to study medicine after being advised in a dream to make him a physician.[2] After a spell in Pergamon as medical officer to the gladiators, Galen went to Rome in 162 and quickly established a large and fashionable practice; the second bloodletting work gives a lively account of how he did it. It was not long before he was attending the emperor Marcus Aurelius, who had, if we can believe Galen, some very complimentary things to say about him.[3] Galen wrote a short work, *That the Best Physician is also a Philosopher*,[4] in which he condemned the ignorant and materialistically-minded doctors of his time, and urged physicians to emulate Hippocrates, who, at least according to Galen, had despised possessions and the pleasures of the table and the bed, and laboured unceasingly in the pursuit of knowledge. Considering the temptations to which he was exposed in Rome, it might perhaps seem surprising that Galen should have followed his own advice to doctors; yet there is good evidence that he did, for with the numbers of patients that he saw, the very extensive research, particularly in anatomy, that he conducted, and the vast quantity of works that he wrote, he could have had very little time for any other activity at all. Many of his writings were destroyed during his lifetime

---

[1] His other names are unknown. There is no evidence for Claudius; it has been suggested that it arose through a misunderstanding of the honorific abbreviation Cl (*clarissimus*, most famous).

[2] For Galen's parents and education see K v, 40ff.; for his father's dream, K x, 609. See also D. E. Eichholz, 'Galen and his environment', *Greece & Rome* 20 (1951) 60–71.

[3] See the work *Prognosis*, K xiv, 657–60. There is a recent critical edition, with English translation, by V. Nutton (*Galen on Prognosis*, 1978). This work of Galen is full of information on social conditions and medical practice in second-century Rome.

[4] K i, 53–63. I have published a translation (*South African Medical Journal* 52 (1977) 936–8).

in a fire; yet in spite of this loss and the depredations of seventeen centuries, Kühn's nineteenth-century edition still runs to twenty-two thick volumes of Greek texts with Latin translations, and some of Galen's other productions survive as versions in Semitic languages. His works extend over anatomy, physiology, medical practice and treatment, prognosis, materia medica, pathology, psychology and psychiatry, the preservation of health, the opinions of the ancients, the medical sects, logic and philosophy. As Nutton has well said, however, they occupy a smaller place in the affections of classicists than on the library shelf;[5] he might have added that this applies even to the edition in microfiche. No one who could have Homer or Sophocles would read Galen for literary enjoyment; his Greek is unattractive and frequently difficult, and to understand the technical side of his writing a background in medicine and science, which few classicists possess, is necessary. But the medical interest and importance of his works is very great; right up to the Renaissance, and long after it in some fields, he was a supreme figure in medicine, and his influence persisted into the nineteenth century and is still very much alive in folk medicine and the metaphors of common speech.

Galen's systems of physiology and pathology are grounded in his concept of nature, which is an unfashionable one in the scientific medicine of today. He has described the differences between two schools of thought in his work *On the Natural Faculties*, in the course of a discussion of nutrition:

Nutrition must involve, therefore, a certain assimilation of nutriment to the thing that is nourished; this is quite clear. Some people, however, maintain that this assimilation does not exist, and is only apparent; they are those who consider that nature is neither craftsmanlike nor providential toward the animal, and that she has no special faculties at all, by which she changes some things, attracts others, and eliminates others again. Two kinds of sects have arisen in medicine and philosophy among those who have declared their views on nature . . . One sect maintains that all substance subject to generation and decay is continuous and subject to change. The other sect supposes substance to be unchangeable, unalterable, and divided into minute particles, separated by regions of empty space . . . According to this second sect, there is no substance or power that is peculiar to nature or mind, but nature and mind are brought about according to the way in which these primary bodies . . . come together. According to the first-mentioned sect, however, nature is not posterior to the atoms, but prior by far and more ancient. And so, in their view, nature herself constructs the bodies both of plants and of animals, using certain faculties that she has, the attractive, the assimilative of what is proper, and the excretory power for getting rid of what is foreign; and she moulds

---

[5] V. Nutton, 'Galen and medical autobiography', *Proc. Camb. Philol. Soc.* 18 (1972) 50–62.

everything in a craftsmanlike manner while it is coming into being, and provides for the finished creatures by means of other powers again.[6]

According to Galen, Hippocrates held this view of a craftsmanlike nature.[7] This is questionable; there is no doubt, however, that Galen did. He saw the bodies of living things as works of art, put together by an intelligent nature with a purpose in mind; members of the atomist school regarded them as having come into existence by chance.[8] Galen alleges, for example, that they thought the mouth had been formed by pneuma or breath bursting out at that place. But why, he asks, if this is so, did it not burst out of the top of the head, since it is characteristic of pneuma to rise to the highest point? And why is the mouth fitted with teeth, beautifully arranged in order like a chorus, and perfectly adapted to perform their function, if it came about by chance? After all, no other cavity in the body has teeth; there are none, for instance, in the rectum or the vagina. It seems, says Galen, that the atoms, which according to the materialist school move at random to form such structures, are behaving more intelligently here than the philosophers who postulate them.[9]

This passage comes from Galen's large work *On the Uses of the Parts*,[10] which, he tells us, he wrote to confute the materialists who did not believe in a purposive and craftsmanlike nature. They used to spend their time, he says, trying to think of just one part of the body that had no purpose.[11] In this work Galen's attitude is profoundly religious; he says that a reverent study of the works of the Creator is more acceptable than costly sacrifices,[12] and that he has written a work that is a perfect theology, a thing far greater and more noble than anything in medicine.[13] In other works his attitude may be less explicitly religious, but he always regards nature as a purposive agent.[14]

[6] K II, 26–7. An English translation of this work by A. J. Brock, *Galen on the Natural Faculties* (Loeb Classical Library, 1916), was for many years the only work of Galen readily available in English.

[7] K II, 29. Galen's attribution of any opinion to Hippocrates must be accepted with extreme caution, since his Hippocrates is a fictitious character who has all Galen's opinions. For a convincing exposition of this thesis, see W. D. Smith, *The Hippocratic tradition* (1979).

[8] For this view see Lucretius II. 1052–66.

[9] K II, 867–74. In his zeal to make his opponents look ridiculous Galen is certainly being unfair to the atomists; one might plead in his defence, however, that it is difficult to see how anyone could have effectively opposed the argument from design in the days before Darwin.

[10] There is an English translation by M. T. May, *Galen on the Usefulness of the Parts of the Body* (2 vols., 1968), with a good account of Galen's physiology.

[11] K IV, 351. [12] K III, 237. [13] K IV, 360.

[14] Galen's works are so voluminous, and what he says in a particular place depends so much on whom he is attacking, the stage of his development, and the state of his

Unlike the God of Moses, however (Galen was neither a Christian nor a Jew), nature is not omnipotent. God has only to ordain something, and it forthwith is; nature must operate according to the ordinary laws of cause and effect, and use whatever material is available. She cannot make a horse or a bull out of ashes.[15] She must take some bodily beginning for the genesis of living things, since she cannot create them out of nothing.[16] Hence, although she is intelligent, she is also intelligible; this makes science possible.

Disease and health, for Galen, are defined in terms of nature. Disease is an unnatural state of the body, which impairs a function; health is a state in accordance with nature, and the cause of the functions.[17] Since nature is purposive and solicitous for the good of the creature, she does her best to restore unnatural states to their healthy condition; this is the famous *vis medicatrix naturae*, of which Galen is the supreme exponent. The function of the physician is to cooperate with her. When a patient is suffering from a disease, nature is struggling to overcome the pathogenic agents,[18] and if she is plainly succeeding the physician should do nothing. If, however, she is getting the worse of the struggle he must come to her aid by doing what she would do if she could. The physician must preserve what is according to nature, eliminate what is not.[19] Galen believes that this was Hippocrates' opinion.[20]

The difference between Galen and the materialists can be seen also in their ideas of causation in biology. For Galen, the important cause is usually what is technically called the final cause: the purpose or end for which something is done. The materialists reject final causes, because they do not believe in a purposive nature.[21] Galen gives an example of a final cause in the actions of a man going to market. If asked why he was going, he would scarcely reply that it was because he had two legs that supported his body and conveyed it over the ground. This is certainly one cause of his actions, an instrumental cause, but the important cause, where a purposive being is involved, is the final one, the man's purpose in going: to buy something, or to meet his friends.[22] Galen attributes final causes to nature because, in his view, she is also an intelligent and purposive agent. She does everything with an aim in mind, and arranges everything in the best

humours at the time, that it is a decidedly rash (though necessary) undertaking to summarise his system in a few pages. The reader must bear in mind that what follows is a considerable over-simplification of Galen's frequently contradictory scheme of pathology.
[15] K III, 906.   [16] K VII, 677.   [17] K VI, 837.   [18] K VII, 194–6.   [19] K x, 589.
[20] K XI, 159–60.   [21] Aristotle, *De resp.* 471b–472a.   [22] K III, 464.

possible way; as both Aristotle and Galen repeatedly say, she does nothing in vain.

This purposive nature operates in bodies through certain faculties or powers (*dynameis*, singular *dynamis*) which she has, on which Galen wrote a special work. Her principal activities are genesis, growth and nutrition.[23] Genesis is concerned with the formation of the embryo. Operating through the semen, which has the alterative faculty, she changes the menstrual blood of the mother, which is retained in the body during pregnancy, into the tissues and organs of the new animal; she is thus cleverer than a human craftsman, like Phidias, who cannot change his wax into gold or ivory. The semen also has an attractive faculty, by which it draws the blood to itself, and a moulding or diaplastic faculty by which it shapes it;[24] this faculty is intensely craftsmanlike and artistic, and does everything for a purpose, so that no part is vain or superfluous, or susceptible of any improvement.[25]

The faculty of growth operates on the parts that have thus come into being, increasing their bulk while retaining their form.[26] The nutritive faculty converts food and drink taken into the body into the parts of the animal, through the medium of the blood, the function of which is to carry nourishment to them. The blood is converted into the tissues of the body, more or less directly in proportion to their similarity to blood. For it to change to flesh is comparatively simple; to make it into bone involves a much longer process. Foods vary, too, in the readiness with which they are convertible into useful blood: blood, that is, that fulfils its proper function, namely to nourish. Meat, in man, can be converted almost completely to useful blood; there is only a small residue, or *perittoma*, that is qualitatively unsuitable for conversion. Man cannot convert grass at all; it is all residue, while a vegetable like the radish has only a small useful component and a great deal of residue. To expel such residues, nature makes use of a further faculty, the eliminative; she absorbs what she wants through her attractive faculty, and eliminates the remainder. Since she is not only craftsmanlike but also solicitous for the good of the animal, she attracts only things that are appropriate.[27]

Galen makes nature rule the body from three centres, the seats of Plato's three parts of the soul; these are the liver, the heart and the brain, which distribute their influence through the veins, arteries and nerves respectively. Galen says that Hippocrates was right in holding this view, rather than the Aristotelian one that all the faculties are

---

[23] K ɪɪ, 10–11. [24] K ɪɪ, 82–6. [25] K ɪɪ, 15. [26] K ɪɪ, 16–17. [27] K ɪɪ, 46.

centred in the heart.[28] The nutritive faculty, also called the appetitive, originates in the liver, which is also the origin of the veins, in which the blood is made from material absorbed from the bowel.[29] This faculty is also concerned with the enjoyment of pleasures. A rather more noble power is distributed through the arteries from its origin in the heart; this is the spirited or vital faculty, and its function is to provide the tone of the soul, to be constant in carrying out the commands of reason, and, in anger, to provide the seething of the innate heat, which is seated in the left ventricle of the heart. It distributes warmth and the ability to grow to all the parts, and endows the arteries with their pulses; the state of this faculty can be judged by feeling the pulse, and gives an indication of what Galen called the strength of the faculty, very important in the successful practice of bloodletting. The most noble faculty of all, the logical, has its seat in the brain, and distributes through the nerves a material known as the psychic pneuma, which is formed in the cerebral ventricles. Thus it confers sensation and voluntary movement on the parts, and provides imagination and memory, knowledge and thought.[30] In Plato's view this was the only part of the soul that was immortal; Galen, although his respect for Plato is second only to that for Hippocrates, is uncertain about the immortality of any of the parts, holding that this is a question for speculative philosophy rather than for medicine.[31]

Nature constructs everything, in the world below the moon, out of the four *elements*, Earth, Water, Air and Fire, which are associated with the four Aristotelian *qualities*, the Hot, the Cold, the Damp and the Dry. Fire is hot and dry; air hot and damp; water cold and damp; and earth cold and dry. In the celestial bodies there is a fifth element, aether, more divine than the materials of the sublunary sphere; it occurs in living creatures, however, in the innate heat of the heart and in the semen, which has the power of generating life just as the sun's heat has. Although Galen wrote a complete work to show that Hippocrates referred to the physical elements,[32] they are of little importance in his medical thought. The four qualities, on the other hand, are vital to it. They are associated, in the bodies of all animals having blood, with four fluids or *humours*, which could thus be thought of as the elements of this kind of living matter. They are

[28] *On the doctrines of Hippocrates and Plato*, ed. P. de Lacy (1980), vol. I, p. 65 (fragment not in Kühn).

[29] K x, 635. It is important to remember that in Galen's system there is no circulation; the flow in both arteries *and veins* is *away from* the centre, and the blood moves slowly outwards in the veins to nourish the body, being replaced at the centre as it is used up at the periphery.

[30] K v, 600–2.   [31] K v, 791–4; K IV, 772–3.

[32] On the *Elements according to Hippocrates*, K I, 413–508.

yellow bile, hot and dry; blood, hot and damp; phlegm, cold and damp; and black bile, cold and dry. The first three are real components of bodies, but black bile is in fact a fictitious substance invented to make up the total of four. Galen took over his humoral system from a work in the Hippocratic corpus, *Nature of Man*,[33] and developed it to expose a mass of contradictions which he was quite unable to reconcile; in spite of this he stuck to it throughout his life, and what is worse, bequeathed it to a long posterity.

The first essential feature of Galen's system, then, is that of a purposive and craftsmanlike nature who creates and regulates the bodies of living things. The second is the principle of balance. The four qualities, and the four humours with which they are associated, have opposite characteristics. Yellow bile and blood contain the Hot, while phlegm and black bile are cold; blood and phlegm are damp, yellow bile and black bile dry. The idea of balance apparently goes back to Alcmaeon of Croton, who held that health consisted in an equal balance of opposites, disease in a preponderance or *monarchia* (Galen does not use the term) of one of them. Both the body and the mind are affected by the balance of the humours, although the developed doctrine of the four mental temperaments, the sanguine, the choleric, the phlegmatic and the melancholic, is post-Galenic. This gives rise to the system of treatment, which Galen says is Hippocratic, by which opposites are the cures for their opposites. If the patient is too hot, he is treated by cooling; if too dry, by dampening, and so on. Health is seen as a harmonious balance of the four qualities, and hence of the four humours, in the body. One of the contradictions in Galen's system becomes apparent here. The two biles and phlegm are pathological humours, in the sense that Galen has great difficulty in deciding what they are there for, except to preserve the balance; yellow bile, for instance, is pathologically hot and dry, and if there is too much of it in the body the result is a fever. If health consists in a perfect mixture or *crasis* – a *eucrasia* – of the four qualities and humours in the body, and disease in a *dyscrasia* or unbalanced mixture, then each of the humours should, when present in excess, be capable of producing such a dyscrasia; they must be, when considered in isolation, essentially dyscrasic. The two varieties of bile, and phlegm, are of this sort, but Galen cannot bring himself to admit it of blood. He compares the four humours to the four seasons of the year, an idea that also comes from *Nature of Man*. Blood corresponds to spring, the season in which it characteristically increases in the body, and in

---

[33] *Nature of Man*, L 6, 32–69, with French translation. There is an English translation by W. H. S. Jones in the Loeb Classical Library, *Hippocrates* vol. IV, pp. 2–41.

Galen's view spring, unlike the other seasons, has to be thought of as eucrasic or well-tempered. It is neither too hot nor too cold, too wet nor too dry; it is temperate in everything.[34] The same applies to blood; after all, the whole nutrition of the body depends on it, and if some malfunction of digestion produces blood that is distempered or dyscrasic, the result is disease. How such a well-tempered humour, with no particular quality in excess, can participate in a scheme of balance with three ill-tempered ones – a well-born hero among three misbegotten villains – is not made clear.

The pathology of internal diseases in Galen's system, though not in several others also fashionable in his time, is largely concerned with dyscrasia. The first level of complexity in living bodies is that of the tissues, or in Galen's and Aristotle's terminology the *homoiomerous parts*; these are substances such as bone, flesh and the humours which have no naked-eye structure. They are formed from the four elements, which however are so mixed in them that none is individually perceptible.[35] Diseases of homoiomerous parts are due to dyscrasia only, since these parts have no structure, if we exclude surgical conditions involving loss of continuity: wounds, ulcers, fractures and so on.

The next level is the organic. Individual organs, such as the arm, are constructed by nature, using the homoiomerous substances as material, just as a human craftsman makes a complicated object from several different homoiomerous materials; for example, gold, silver and ivory. Thus the arm consists of blood, flesh, skin, vein, nerve, etc., all arranged by nature to ensure the best possible performance of its function. Disease of an organ, then, may be due to dyscrasia or to loss of continuity in any of its homoiomerous components, sufficient to impair the function of the organ; it may also, however, result from some defect of structure, or in Galen's term *diaplasis*, arising during the formation of the body from the maternal blood under the influence of the diaplastic or moulding faculty, or subsequently from trauma or some such cause. Such a structural abnormality, though unnatural, amounts to disease only if it appreciably impairs the function of the organ.[36]

Although Galen pays lip service to the four qualities as equal opposites, for him, as probably for Aristotle, the most important one is the Hot. There are two kinds of heat; the ordinary variety, which burns things up, and the *innate heat* of living creatures, which makes the body grow instead of consuming it, and also has the power of generation. The innate heat is often equated with nature in Galen's

---

[34] K xv, 88. See also K i, 524–34.   [35] K xv, 7–8; K i, 467–8.   [36] K x, 125–6.

works; it is the life of the body, which dies when it is extinguished. Since it is distributed to every part with the arterial blood, it is often also equated with blood. The innate heat, as its name suggests, is not acquired from outside; it comes to the embryo through the semen, which contains the hot principle, and resides in the arterial blood of the left ventricle when the heart is formed. The function of respiration is to moderate the intensity of the innate heat in the left heart; pneuma or breath derived from inspired air is mixed with the arterial blood in the left heart, and distributed with it. Respiration, in the form of transpiration, also takes place through the open distal ends of the arteries, which communicate through pores in the skin with the outside air. As the arterial blood alternately advances and recedes with the movement of the pulse, the smoky residues of combustion in the heart are alternately discharged through the pores and fresh air drawn in.[37]

The innate heat is most abundant at birth, and since it is in the blood, babies have, relatively speaking, more blood than adults; Galen remarks that even their bones show it.[38] In old age both the heat and the amount of blood are greatly reduced; hence Lady Macbeth's surprise that the old man should have so much blood in him.[39] As a result, the young are more liable to hot diseases, the fevers, and the old to cold ones such as palsies and coryzas.

Although the innate heat is a special kind of heat, and is not derived from any outside source, it is augmented by nourishment that the body can use, just as adding fuel, in moderation, augments the heat of a fire. Of all articles of food, wine, taken in moderation, increases the innate heat most effectively; in excess, however, it has the opposite effect.[40]

One of the most important functions of the innate heat is to preside over pepsis or digestion, the conversion of food and drink in the gut into useful blood. This conversion takes place in what Galen called the first veins – the modern portal system – and the veins in the liver. Perfectly pure blood does not exist in the body, just as unmixed elements are not found on earth; it always has some admixture of the other three humours. In useful blood, which provides the best nourishment to the tissues of the body, no particular quality prevails;

[37] For the innate heat, see K vii, 616–18; for respiration, K iv, 471–83, and D. J. Furley and J. S. Wilkie, *Galen on respiration and the arteries* (1984) in which the relevant works are translated.

[38] K xviiia, 238. Unlike adults, babies have red (haemopoietic) marrow in the shafts of the long bones.

[39] *Macbeth* v, 1. Shakespeare makes the aged Nestor say 'I'll prove this truth with my three drops of blood' (*Troilus and Cressida* i, 3).

[40] K i, 659–61.

it is well tempered or balanced. For blood of this kind to be produced, the amount of heat applied to the digestive process must be exactly right. The Greek word *pepsis*, and its equivalent from the Latin, coction, mean cooking or ripening.[41] If too much heat is applied, and the blood is overcooked, it will contain too much of the hot humour, yellow bile, and the patient may become feverish; if there is too little heat, on the other hand, there will be too much phlegm in the cold and insufficiently cooked blood. Neither kind can nourish as well as the perfectly eucrasic blood that results from the application of exactly the right amount of heat. From the liver, the root of the veins in Galen's system, the venous blood is distributed to the periphery through the veins, except for some that goes to the right side of the heart. From here on, one portion of it goes to the lungs, to nourish them; the remainder passes through the interventricular septum by impercept-ible pores, and is combined in the left ventricle with pneuma from the lungs to make the arterial blood, with which the innate heat from the left ventricle is distributed to the parts to make them grow. There is no good evidence that Galen knew of the pulmonary circulation, or any circulation of the blood at all.

Both the veins and the arteries form branching systems, reaching to every part of the body; they end in minute orifices, normally imper-meable to blood, distributed over the entire body surface. At least according to Erasistratus, Galen's opponent in the first two bloodlet-ting works, communications or inosculations existed between veins and arteries near their distal ends, though these were normally closed; in his view the arteries in life contained pneuma but no blood, and inflammation was due to the passage across into the ends of the arteries of blood from the veins, when the pneuma in the arteries had been allowed to escape as a result of trauma.[42] Galen wrote a special work, and undertook experiments, to show that there actually was blood in the arteries in the living animal.[43]

Too much heat in the body may result in a fever, of which there are several varieties. In Galen's system all fevers are pathological dyscra-sias of the Hot; he would not have agreed with the modern idea, which some of the ancients seem to have held also, that fever is a beneficial adaptation. There are several ways, in Galen's system, in which the body can become hotter than it should, suffering, in his words, 'the unnatural heat which we call fever'.[44] Fever occurs when the heat increases to such an immoderate degree as to distress the patient and

---

[41] For digestion, see K xv, 596–7; K ɪɪ, 163–4.
[42] For Erasistratus and his pathology, see K xɪ, 153–4 (below, pp. 18–20) and p. 16 n.6.
[43] K ɪv, 703–36.   [44] K vɪɪ, 277.

damage a function. If there is no functional impairment, the patient is merely hot, not feverish. Since all fevers are, by definition, against nature, they all need treatment with a damp and cold regimen unless there is some contra-indication.[45]

Galen, unlike some of the ancients whom he cites, postulated more than one mechanism for fever. The simplest variety, which he calls the ephemeral (though it may last longer than a day), is due simply to overheating of the body by the sun, anger, exertion, heat-producing foods or drinks, or to reduction of heat loss through insufficient transpiration when the pores of the skin are obstructed.[46] Other fevers are the result of inflammation, with or without putrefaction. Both inflammation and putrefaction originate from residues, or peritto-mata, in the body, which are thus extremely important in Galen's pathology.

Residues accumulate when more nourishment is taken in than the body requires. Although these surplus products of digestion are always mixtures of humours, they are classified according to the humour that predominates. An excess characterised by yellow bile, black bile or phlegm constitutes a *cacochymia*; a superfluity of blood, on the other hand, is called a *plethos* or *plethora*, from the Greek for abundance. This is because blood, as previously mentioned, is not a pathological humour. Plethos, however, may be a pathological state; it is possible to have too much even of a good thing, and this is one of the principal indications for bloodletting. The perittomatous accumu-lations of humours move about in the body, flowing (hence the term *fluxion*) into various parts. The natural excretory faculty in the affected part, however, will push the residue out of it if it is strong enough to do so; the flux of humours will then look elsewhere for a home in a part whose excretory faculty is too feeble to eject it, and when it finds one it will settle down in it and establish a focus of inflammation. Diseases due to such a descent of humours on a part are rheumatic in the old, wider sense; the derivation is from *rheo*, I flow, and the term applies to all conditions with this aetiology, whether or not the affected part is a joint. Thus the parts with the feeblest excretory powers are the ones most likely to provide hospitality for wandering residues; for example the skin, lymph nodes (which Galen calls the glands) and the brain. The brain, however, is a fortunate organ in that it is provided with passages leading downward through which the humours can escape; they descend from the ventricles through the holes in the cribriform plate and out at the nose, or escape from other parts of the head.[47]

[45] K x, 532, 589.   [46] For ephemeral fevers, see K x, 665–7; K vii, 296–7, 302.
[47] For residues and their movements, see translation K xi, 275–6.

The nature of the inflammatory condition in the part affected by a rheumatic process depends both on the part and on the humour concerned. If it is phlegm, it will produce a watery swelling; yellow bile leads to ulceration, black bile to scirrhous tumours, and an excess of heated blood to the classical signs of inflammation.[48] Such an excess of blood, or plethos, can be of two kinds, concerning which Galen wrote a complete work[49] to instruct the doctors of his time, whose only response to his questions on the subject, he says, was a vacant fishlike stare. This is a complicated doctrine, which leaves the reader in some doubt whether Galen himself understood it completely; he has not told us what its effect on the physicians was. In brief, there are two kinds of plethos: dynamic plethos (*pros dynamin*), and a variety *pros to enchyma*, which I translate 'plethos by filling'. The dynamic variety is due to the weakness of the dynamis, here the excretory faculty, in the part concerned; the essential thing about it is not so much the excessive quantity of humour as the inability of the part to expel it. The variety called plethos by filling is due to the distension of the vessels by the excess, which may rupture them. This variety has the more mechanical causation, and it can occur even in inanimate containers such as wine-jars. In the dynamic variety the natural faculties are burdened, and the chief symptom is a feeling of weight and sluggishness; in plethos by filling the patient feels distended.[50]

The heat resulting from a flux of hot humours to a part can spread by contiguity until it reaches the heart, and when the heart is overheated the result is a fever, since the heat will be distributed to every part of the body. The second main variety of fever, then, occurs as a result of simple inflammation in some part, the heat from which has extended to the heart. There is a grave danger, however, that perittomatous fluxes, once established in a part, may putrefy. When this happens a greater amount of heat is generated, since it is well known that rotting matter becomes hot, and it spreads in the same way; if it reaches the heart, the result is a putrefactive fever.[51]

Putrefactive fevers are particularly likely to occur when damp and hot conditions, such as promote rotting, prevail. When the body is in this state, and is full of residues as a result of overindulgence, it is likely to provide a fertile soil for seeds of contagion if they are present in the atmosphere. Epidemic diseases are caused in this way; hence the injunction in *Nature of Man* to keep the body as thin and weak as

---

[48] Galen wrote a special work on abnormal swellings, K vii, 705–32. There is an English translation by D. G. Lytton and L. M. Resuhr, *J. Hist. Med.* 33 (1978) 531–49.

[49] K vii, 513–83.   [50] See translation, K xi, 258–61.

[51] See translation, K xi, 262–5.

possible in times of pestilence.[52] Galen's idea of seeds of pestilence in the air is an interesting anticipation of the nineteenth-century germ theory of disease; it goes back to the Hippocratic corpus.

The last distinction that must be drawn is that between fevers due to anomalous dyscrasias, and the hectic fevers. Galen wrote a special work on the anomalous dyscrasias. In brief, the body suffers an anomalous dyscrasia when one part of it is unnaturally hotter, or colder, or wetter, or drier, than another; if the dyscrasic process spreads so that the whole body is uniformly involved, it is no longer anomalous. Now since pain, and indeed every symptom, is due to change (or motion in the Aristotelian sense), once the body is uniformly affected by the pathological process there will be no symptoms; as the patient is equally hot all over, he does not feel hot at all, although he is suffering from the most dangerous of fevers, the hectic variety. Such fevers have no periodicity.[53] Galen does his best to account for the periodicity of some of the other varieties of fever by a consideration of the rotting and spontaneous combustion of pigeon droppings, but has no convincing explanation to offer.[54]

In Galen's view, then, there are three main kinds of fever. The ephemeral variety is due merely to temporary overheating of the body; the cause is no longer operating, and the doctor's only task is to cool it. The inflammatory fevers are more difficult; here it may be necessary to dissipate the inflammatory focus, and bloodletting is one of the possible measures. If, however, the flux of humours to a part has gone on to putrefy, his problems are multiplied, since measures that inhibit putrefaction may increase the fever,[55] probably because local cooling remedies decrease transpiration. Hence the extreme importance, in the ancient system, of keeping the body free from residues in the first place; constipation, or the suppression of a menstrual period, was regarded as a very serious matter because material that ought to be got rid of was being retained in the body, and much attention was given to prophylaxis. The idea is by no means dead in popular belief even today.

The principal indication for bloodletting, then, is to eliminate such residues, or to prevent them from accumulating in the first place. Another is to divert blood from one part to another by the process known as revulsion or derivation. If the patient is bleeding to death from one part of the body, open a vein in another, and the bleeding

---

[52] K vii, 291–3, 295. The remark in *Nature of Man* is at L 6, 54–6; see also Celsus 1.10.1. For contagion, see V. Nutton, 'The seeds of disease; an explanation of contagion and infection from the Greeks to the Renaissance', *Med. Hist.* 27 (1983) 1–34.

[53] *On Anomalous Dyscrasias*, K vii, 733–52.   [54] K i, 657–8; K vii, 298–9, 379–90.

[55] K x, 661–3.

from the first will stop.[56] The advantage of bloodletting over other sorts of haemorrhage, as Galen repeatedly says, is that the doctor can stop the flow whenever he wishes.

Galen's system of pathology, although sometimes complicated in its details, is in principle very simple. All medical diseases are due to dyscrasia of one sort or another, and all that the doctor has to do is to restore the balance of the humours in the body. His task is made difficult, however, because individual patients differ greatly in their natural crases. Some are by nature cold, and hence more liable to conditions like dropsy than to fevers; others are hot, and so on. It is of great practical importance to judge the natural crasis, or temperament, of the patient. This is not a simple matter, however, since different parts of the patient may have different temperaments; neither is treatment by rule of thumb possible, since every patient must be assessed individually in terms both of his natural temperament and physical type and of his way of life, past and present.[57] Here Galen differs notably from simplifiers such as the Methodist sect, who had only one rule for all. None the less, his system is, by modern standards, simple, and at first sight logical; no one could accuse him of a reductionist approach. Galen's one grand unified theory will account for everything in medicine.

[56] For revulsion see, e.g. K xi, 178–9 (p. 33 below); also M.-H. Marganne, 'Sur l'origine hippocratique des concepts de révulsion et de dérivation', *L'Antiquité classique* 49 (1980) 115–30.

[57] Perhaps Galen's most famous work, the *Techne Iatrike* or *Ars Medica* (Tegni Galeni in dog-Latin) is largely concerned with this practical problem. It tells the doctor how to judge the crasis of the patient or any part of him, from his physical and psychological characteristics. There is no modern English translation; the Greek is in K i, 305–412.

++

CHAPTER 2

Galeni de Venae Sectione adversus Erasistratum Liber
Galen's Book on Venesection against Erasistratus

The first chapter of the second bloodletting work (pp. 38–42 below) explains that this first book is a verbatim transcript of an address by Galen to a gathering of philosophers, in which he attacked Erasistratus. It was taken down, he says, at the request of a friend who wanted it for his private use, and was never intended for wider distribution.

It seems to me to be a question well worth investigating, why on earth Erasistratus,[1] who was, after all, so competent in the other branches of the Art, and so meticulous about the minutest detail as to describe even the boiling of certain vegetables and of plasters – matters on which it would have sufficed any one else just to say what was essential and to omit the mode of preparation, as a minor point which anyone could pick up as he went along – why Erasistratus, in the case of such a powerful and important remedy as phlebotomy, and one that was esteemed by the ancients as in no way inferior to the most effective of all, has nothing to say.[2] The fact is that the word K148 phlebotomy is scarcely to be found in any work of his; the one exception is in his book on bringing up blood,[3] but even here he mentions it more, it would seem, in passing than as something he was considering with the care it deserves. You can see this from his actual words, which are as follows:

---

[1] Erasistratus of Ceos practised in Alexandria in the third century BC, about 400 years before Galen. His works are lost except for fragments quoted by other writers. There was still a strong Erasistratean sect in Rome in Galen's time; hence the effort Galen expends in attacking him. The opinions of Erasistratus, or at any rate Galen's version of them, will appear in the course of the work. See J. F. Dobson, 'Erasistratus', *Proc. Roy. Soc. Med.* part 3 (1927) 825–32; I. M. Lonie, 'Erasistratus, the Erasistrateans, and Aristotle', *Bull. Hist. Med.* 38 (1964) 426–43; G. E. R. Lloyd, 'A note on Erasistratus of Ceos', *J. Hellen. Stud.* 95 (1975) 172–5; L. G. Wilson, 'Erasistratus, Galen and the pneuma', *Bull. Hist. Med.* 33 (1959) 293–314; W. D. Smith, 'Erasistratus's dietetic medicine', *Bull. Hist. Med.* 56 (1982) 398–409; P. M. Fraser, *Ptolemaic Alexandria* (1972) vol. I, pp. 347–9.

[2] Galen's opening sentence would do credit to *Tristram Shandy*. Its structure has been preserved in the translation, although elsewhere such elaborate passages have sometimes been broken up for ease of comprehension.

[3] αἵματος ἀναγωγή, translated 'bringing up blood' since it includes both haemoptysis and haematemesis; the former is meant here.

15

'Bandages should be applied at the armpits and groins, not in the manner of some imitators of the treatment, who do not realise that it is done for the sake of the blood, but rather squeezing it out thoroughly with the ligatures.[4] A considerable amount of blood is sequestrated in the bandaged parts of the limbs, as both the distension of the veins and phlebotomy show. It flows far more copiously when bandages are applied to the part of the body in which the vein is opened. In patients who bring up blood, most of the blood should be cut off[5] by bindings on the legs and arms, since with the reduction in the amount of blood in the region of the chest, the ejection of blood will be alleviated. It is this same effect that the phlebotomists wish to achieve in patients who bring up blood. Chrysippus, however, is far better, since he does not consider only

K149   the present, but takes impending dangers into account as well. Bringing up blood is dangerous because the danger of inflammation is linked with it, and in the presence of inflammation the nutrition of the patient presents a problem; a patient who has been phlebotomised in addition to being kept long without food is in danger of fainting. But Chrysippus, who transfers nourishment that has already been prepared in the body to unaffected parts, and will bring it back in the same way at the time when fainting threatens, thus making use of nutriment that is already there and not being compelled to administer food, is altogether pre-eminent in understanding and worthy of praise, and entirely self-consistent.'[6]

It is clear to anyone that these are insignificant and random observations, worthy neither of Erasistratus' expertise in the Art nor of the power of the remedy. If no description of it were to be found in the works of Hippocrates, Diocles or Euryphon,[7] or in those of any of

---

4 Literally 'but they squeeze it out sufficiently with the bandages'. The meaning seems to be that the ignorant practitioners apply the bandages too loosely to squeeze the blood into the extremities. For Erasistratus' bandaging method see also Celsus IV.11.7.

5 Reading αἵματος δεῖ πλεῖστον ἀπολαμβανεσθαι with A, U and M.

6 Erasistratus believed that inflammation, and the fever resulting from it, was due to the passing across of blood from the veins into the arteries; since feeding filled the veins with new blood, which impeded the healing passage of blood back into the veins from the arteries, it was important not to feed the patient when inflammation threatened. The sequestration of blood in the extremities at this time thus had a dual value; it reduced the likelihood of inflammation developing in the chest, and at the same time made it possible to release some of the blood whenever desired, to nourish the patient who was receiving nothing by mouth. Little is known of Erasistratus' teacher Chrysippus who developed this treatment; he is not the Stoic of that name. Several Chrysippi, one of whom he may have been, are mentioned in Fraser, vol. I, p. 347; vol. II, p. 502. His method is an interesting anticipation of the modern practice of auto-transfusion, and the antithesis of the even more modern medical antishock trousers, which squeeze blood out of the legs so that the vital centres get more of it.

7 The so-called works of Hippocrates (the Hippocratic corpus or collection) are obviously the productions of several different authors and periods, from the fifth to the

Erasistratus' predecessors at all, one might well think that he had disregarded it with good reason, since it had never been found useful or held in esteem by the most eminent men. But since, in fact, other references to it are to be found, and there was already some consider- K150 able use of the remedy, not only in one disease or an unimportant one, but in the majority and the most acute; and since Hippocrates himself, whom we regard as the leader of all the distinguished men in the profession, and the other men of old clearly did use it; what ever then has come over Erasistratus, that he has totally neglected to discuss it in any detail? Indeed, if he approved of it, he ought to indicate this by describing the conditions for which it was appropriate, as he does with the other remedies; if it pleased him, he ought to say why. But he is so reluctant to show his hand in the matter of the efficacy of the remedy, that he does not indicate whether it should be used or not used, and does not dare to reveal what opinion he holds except once, as I said, in connection with one disease. And yet the gist of his opinion is manifest even from the occasions on which he says nothing; for surely he would not have disregarded venesection if he had approved of it, nor considered it necessary to describe insignificant things that were useful in the treatment of diseases, while assuming that anyone would be able to discover such an important one as bloodletting for himself, without any instruction from Erasistratus.[8]

third centuries BC; it is doubtful whether any of them can be attributed with certainty to Hippocrates, of whom we know next to nothing with certainty except that he was a physician of Cos. Galen makes such attributions quite uncritically, although there are some famous works, such as *On Ancient Medicine* and *On The Sacred Disease*, which he never mentions at all, from which we may conclude that, if he knew them, he did not think they were by Hippocrates. There is no complete translation in English; Littré's complete nineteenth-century edition offers one in French. The name Hippocrates, used without qualification in this work, must be understood to mean the author of the work in the Corpus under discussion at the time, just as we say 'Homer' when 'the author of the tenth book of the *Iliad*' would be more correct.

Diocles of Carystos lived in Athens in the fourth century BC; according to one authority, Erasistratus' system was based on his medicine and the physics of Straton (W. Jaeger, *Diokles von Karystos* (1963), p. 227). This is Straton the peripatetic, important for his views on the void or vacuum (see *OCD*, Straton (1); Fraser, vol. I, p. 427), and almost certainly not the medical Straton mentioned in the next chapter. Little is known of Euryphon of Cnidus.

[8] Caelius Aurelianus, a Roman writer probably of the third century AD, says (*CD* II.183) that Erasistratus did use venesection as a revulsive to stop haemorrhage, although some of his followers condemned it on the grounds that it impaired the strength. If this was so, Galen certainly did not know it. For the refutation of another suggestion that Erasistratus approved of it, see F. Kudlien, 'A new testimony for Erasistratus?', *Clio Medica* 15 (1981) 137–42. Another subject on which Erasistratus, according to Galen, had nothing at all to say, was black bile (K v, 104–5, 123). Julian the Methodist, another recipient of Galen's ire for not believing in it, obviously thought that Hippocrates had invented this imaginary humour, since he said that those who praised Hippocrates had been made insane by black bile. This is fighting talk where Galen comes from (K XVIIIa, 291–2).

2. To tell the truth, it might seem that one would need second sight
K151 to discover why he did not use phlebotomy; for how could we know
the views of Erasistratus on matters that he has never referred to in
any detail? None the less, some have been so rash as to try to divine his
opinions; but they are manifestly in error, and one of the chief proofs
of this is in the things in which they differ from one another. Not one
of them thinks the same as the others; and the worst of all is that the
fellow-students of Erasistratus do not agree with the pupils of Chrysippus the Cnidian, the very man who originated the dogma that
phlebotomy should not be used. Not only is there no agreement
whatever among these folk concerning the opinions of Chrysippus,
but the utterances of Apoimantus and of Straton are laughable. They
say that it is a nuisance to have to open a vein, and to make sure that it
is in fact a vein rather than an artery, which, if cut instead of a vein,
may lead to unfortunate consequences. A further difficulty is that
some patients have died of fear, some even before the vessel was cut,
some through never recovering consciousness after the venesection.
Others, again, have bled uncontrollably. Then we have the utterances
K152 of others, some of whom say that it is difficult to estimate the amount
of the evacuation, so that one is compelled either to do no good to the
patient who is insufficiently evacuated, or to cause the gravest harm to
the one in whom the amount is exceeded; for what is the difference,
they say, between unregulated phlebotomy and murder? Others,
again, maintain that an inrush of pneuma into the veins might take
place from the arteries, since pneuma must follow of necessity
through the inosculations when the blood is emptied out.[9] Still others
say that since the inflammatory condition arises in the arteries, there is
no point in emptying the veins. Even if such pronouncements might
seem convincing to some, yet in relation to the truth itself they carry
no conviction and are plainly false. People who express such opinions
would be far more convincing if they said what some other people,
impelled by the nature of the humours, have said. Perhaps one ought
to make an even more extensive criticism of them, but this is not the
time for it, since it would be necessary to draw out the argument to
great lengths. In any case, there is nothing, either in the remarks of
Erasistratus or of any of the other disciples of Chrysippus, to impel
one to undertake such a refutation now.

K153   **3.** I think the best way of arranging my argument would be to omit
the other matters and start with the opinions of Erasistratus himself;

---

[9] This is the opposite of Erasistratus' view (see below, section 3) that blood from the
veins went across to the arteries when the pneuma they normally contained had
escaped through a wound.

they will be dealt with as briefly as possible. He believes that the artery is the vessel of the pneuma, and the vein of the blood. The larger vessels, according to him, repeatedly split up into channels of lesser size but greater number, extending throughout the body – for there is no place where the end of a vessel is not situated – finally forming such minute terminations that by the closing of the mouths at their ends the blood is prevented from escaping and is retained inside them. As a result, although the mouths of the vein and of the artery lie alongside one another, the blood remains within its proper bounds and nowhere encroaches upon the vessels of the pneuma. While this state of affairs continues, the animal is under the rule of a natural process.[10] When, however, some violent cause diverts the blood from the veins into the arteries, disease must necessarily ensue forthwith. He believes further that there are other causes, the most important of which is an excess of blood, which has the dual effect of distending the coat of the vein and of forcing open the ends of the vessels which were previously closed, so that the blood passes across to the arteries and thus collides with the pneuma sent along from the heart and gets in its way, changing some- K154 what[11] the movement of the pneuma when it gets near it and on the side of its origin; this is the condition of fever. Further, he thinks that it is driven forwards by the pneuma and impacted into the ends of the arteries, and that this constitutes inflammation. According to this theory, where there is plethos the result is inflammation. In wounds he also implicates inflammation, in which there is a passing across of blood from the veins into the arteries; but the reason for this passing across, he says, is that the blood is following to fill up an empty space. For when, as the result of a wound, all the pneuma is poured out from the lacerated arteries in the injured part, and there is danger that an empty space will result, the blood follows along the inosculations to fill up the site of the pneuma that has been emptied out.[12] So, when

---

[10] I.e. not a disease, which is against nature.

[11] Reading ἀλλοιοῦν τι. The MSS are of no help, as none of them leaves spaces between words. Ch, like K, has no space, and Ald is doubtful.

[12] According to Galen, Erasistratus accepts only this principle of refilling of a vacuum (see above, n. 7 for his master Straton); he does not accept the natural faculties, one of which is the attractive. Galen says that very thin people, if they are to be made fat, must incorporate more nutriment than corresponds to what they have lost, and this requires that the parts concerned must actively attract the nutriment they require through their attractive faculty (see above, p. 5). If the only mechanism was the refilling of a vacuum, they could never become fatter than they had been in the past (K II, 103–4). Erasistratus, however, believes that all distribution (*anadosis*) of nutriment through the veins is effected by refilling; as nutriment is used up at the periphery, it is replaced so that a vacuum does not develop. He does not say how urine is secreted; according to Galen, this cannot be explained by refilling (K II, 63–4). For the further opinions of Erasistratus on *paremptosis*, the passing across of blood from the veins to the arteries, see Galen's work *On Black Bile*, K v, 125. Galen accepts

the vessel of the pneuma has been opened, the blood[13] is poured out; but when it is stopped and closed, the blood is compressed inside it by the pneuma sent along subsequently by the heart, and all crowded back into the parts round the wound, and inflammation is brought about in this way.

Very well, then; we shall agree, for the present at least, that everything he says about fevers and inflammations is correct, although I have shown in other works that nothing he says of these matters is K155 true; next let him instruct us on the remedies. He speaks, both in many other works and in his third book on fevers, word for word as follows:

'Round about the time, then, at which illnesses are beginning and of the onset of inflammatory conditions, all sloppy foods should be withdrawn.'

and

'The inflammations that give rise to fevers arise for the most part as a result of plethora. So if nourishment is given at such times and digestion and distribution perform their functions, the vessels are filled with nutriment, and more powerful inflammations will ensue.'

So much for the inflammations that originate from plethos in the absence of trauma. As for those that arise from wounds, again in his first book on fevers he says something like this:

'Systems of treatment follow these principles to keep all wounds free from inflammation. The drugs that are rubbed into the surrounding healthy parts prevent, by their styptic and astringent action, the development of pressure[14] by the blood poured out from above on the wounded parts. In the unaffected parts, on the other hand, there comes about an interchange between the many arteries and veins that have inosculations in the same places, transferring to K156 the veins some of the blood that had gone across to the arteries. The practice of not giving food to wounded patients, during the time when inflammation is occurring, is also consistent with these principles; for the veins, when emptied of nutriment, will more readily receive back the blood that has gone across to the arteries, and when this happens the inflammation will become less.'

the principle of refilling (K ɪɪ, 206), but requires the natural faculty of attraction as well.

13 K's text is corrupt, and none of the MSS is of help. That it is the blood that is poured out when the artery is opened seems clear from the next phrase; it can only be the blood that is compressed by the pneuma sent along subsequently. The Latin translator in Ju agrees with me, though the one in K thinks the reference is to pneuma.

14 Reading σύνωσιν, suggested by an examiner, for K's σύνιωσιν. A, U and M have συνενωσιν. K's Latin translator renders it 'impetum'.

Thus far this practice supports the contention of Erasistratus that one ought to evacuate the plethos, and that the veins cannot receive back the blood into themselves if they are filled and distended. The only question is in what way they should be evacuated.

4. I have always thought that once evacuation has been decided on, the easiest and promptest course of action is to open a vein. In this way we would evacuate the actual inflammatory matters themselves, and nothing else; whereas fasting, apart from the long time it requires, evacuates the whole system indiscriminately, and this is not called for. Why should one evacuate what does not need evacuation, and why should one waste the flesh when it is possible to let some blood? I shall pass over the other evils which cannot but follow prolonged fasting: K157 the exhausted strength, the humours becoming bilious and painful, the severe heartburn, nausea and constipation, and all the residues becoming extremely acrid and malignant;[15] yet Erasistratus sees none of these, like blind men, who although a smooth, broad and direct road is near, often take a narrow, rough and long one, and go by a circuitous route. He too, when a short enough way is thus at hand, and one free from trouble, has disregarded it, and travelled instead by a long and difficult one. He considers only one thing, whether the road will get him where he wants to go, and thinks no further whether it will do so quickly and without trouble. Fasting, I grant you, does indeed lead to the evacuation of plethos, but it takes a long time and is accompanied by great distress. In spite of this, however, the sapient Erasistratus, whom some have thought fit to compare with Hippocrates, ignores so great a remedy, and, unabashed at having nothing convincing and reasonable to say, mentions it as if he were speaking of something of very slight importance and no value. But Hippocrates did not take this view of phlebotomy, O Erasistratus, and he was in no way a worse physician than you are. What you applaud in theory is K158 found in him put into practice. You marvel at nature, as something craftsmanlike[16] and at the same time providential towards the living creature; but nowhere do you imitate her. Why is it, if this is not so, that although you have often seen nature healing diseases by evacuation of blood, you have never yet practised it, even in a single one? And why have you nothing to say about the works of the nature whom you praise? Why, when you can find many things like this in Hippocrates: 'A woman vomiting blood cured by the menses breaking

---

15 Reading, with A, U and M, δριμύτερα τε και κακοηθεστερα, as did K's Latin translator.
16 Erasistratus, Galen tells us in another work, though maintaining that nature was craftsmanlike, contradicted himself over and over; he held that the spleen and the renal arteries had no function (K II, 91) and that bile was useless (K II, 78).

out';[17] 'Haemorrhoids protect likewise against black bile';[18] 'Copious haemorrhages from the nostrils are for the most part curative',[19] are there none in your works, but your praise of nature goes no further than lip service, and you write nothing anywhere about the work of nature? For me, the study of nature's works is all that I require; with this for inspiration, I would be able to discover the right course of action. But as for you, I don't suppose your admirers will concede that my remarks are well founded if I say that you appear either to be completely devoid of understanding or to have paid scant attention to K159 the works of nature. You are guilty on one count or the other; either of total ignorance of them, or of understanding but refusing to emulate them. You must have written these things shut up in some house, never seeing a single patient; this is probably why you are ignorant of the works of nature. You are always marvelling but never imitating, which makes you stupid in the last degree.[20]

If, then, you had made up your mind to try your hand at writing – and, I may say, you break the rules of composition when you do – you ought to have first explained to us the operations of nature, and then described the things, on the one hand, that she brings perfectly to a conclusion, when activated by her own laws; and on the other those that she does imperfectly, when she is impeded by the factors that cause diseases. This, after all, is the way to discovery in therapeutics: to be able, through a study of the cases she brings well to a conclusion, to assist the other patients by making good whatever she lacks. And indeed when she is showing no activity at all – a thing that sometimes happens when she is overcome by the strength of the noxious causative agents – we must provide everything ourselves; but you have expounded none of these matters. The reason, I suppose, is that, as they say, you paid little attention to examining patients, but stayed at home and wrote down mere opinions. Even, however, if you did not see patients yourself, you might at least have read the works of Hippocrates, and learned how many cases nature, when she has been set in motion, brings to a crisis perfectly and faultlessly, and, as that K160 man used to say, fittingly; and how, again, one may best imitate her when she is not attempting a crisis; and how, when she is, but is not sufficiently active, one should assist her. If you were trained in these

---

[17] L 4, 542; L 6, 152.   [18] L 4, 566.   [19] Probably L 4, 530.

[20] The text is probably corrupt, but as it stands this is uncalled for. According to Celsus (Prooem, 23–4), Erasistratus dissected living men, and Caelius Aurelianus says that in hepatic disease he used to open the abdomen and pack drugs round the liver (*CD* III.65). These activities, though eccentric, are scarcely those of an armchair philosopher. For Erasistratus' anatomical researches, see Lloyd; Smith (1979) p. 195; Fraser, vol. II, p. 507.

matters I would hear you recommending, as I do Hippocrates, 'not to disturb patients when they are at, or have just passed, the crisis, or to experiment with purgatives or other irritants, but to let them alone'.[21] This is his advice to you when nature is perfectly activated. He goes on to recommend that when nature is moving towards a crisis, but not actively enough, you should assist her: 'Whatever material needs to be led off, evacuate in the direction in which it chiefly tends, through the appropriate passages.'[22] For nature at that time wishes to eject the noxious matter; but when, because of weakness, she cannot bring the work to a conclusion, she needs our help. Applying the principle to the treatment of pleurisy, one should evacuate in the direction in which the humours tend. How does he put it?

'If the pain is in the region of the clavicle, or there is heaviness in the arm, or in the region of the breasts, or above the diaphragm, one should cut the inner vein at the bend of the elbow, and not hesitate K161 to withdraw blood in quantity as long it has a distinctly redder colour as it flows, or is livid instead of being clear and red; for either may occur. If, however, the pain is below the diaphragm, and does not point in the direction of the clavicle, you should soften the bowels either with black hellebore or with peplium.'[23]

Again, where in speaking of a certain combination of nephritic symptoms he says: 'and severe pain in the region of the kidney, numbness of the thigh on the corresponding side', he adds 'cut the ham',[24] that is, open the vein at the back of the thigh.

5. How has he expressed it?

'There was no bleeding from the servant of Stymargos when she gave birth to a daughter; the cervix uteri was retroverted; pain in the hip and leg, relieved by venesection alongside the ankle, although the whole body was involved in shivering.[25] But one must come to the cause and the nourishment of the cause.'[26]

So Hippocrates orders you to enquire into the cause and the origin of the cause. In this connection, I think, you could not say anything else but that when a plethos of blood is causing trouble, venesection must

---

[21] L 4, 468; see also L 2, 50–2. [22] L 4, 468. [23] L 2, 272–4.
[24] Reading νάρκη for K's ἀρχή; Galen is quoting L 5, 268. A, U, and M are all faulty, A with a crux in the margin, but Ch is correct; it is strange that Kühn did not pick this up.
[25] Reading, with A, τρομοι το σωμα παν κατειχον.
[26] L 5, 126. As often elsewhere, K's eccentric punctuation has been disregarded. Littré, probably correctly, makes πρὸς ἰσχίον καὶ σκέλος apply to the pain, not the retroversion; Galen, however, refers it to the uterus on the next page. The word meaning 'origin' was τροφή in Galen's MS of Hippocrates; this is clear since he repeats it on the next page of K. In Littré's text it is ἀρχή, which makes better sense; Galen finds it necessary to explain this meaning of τροφή at K xi, 162, and paraphrases it as γένεσις here. Both K's Latin translator and Ju render the word in question *fomes*.

be ordered.[27] Accordingly, in the case of the above-mentioned woman, although she was suffering a rigor, he did not hesitate to open K162 a vein, although no one else would have dared to remove blood during rigors, just as they would not attempt it in dropsy or any other cold condition. The reason is that in such cases it might be expected to cool the body still more as a result of the removal of the warm humour, and extinguish the innate heat, which had already been cooled by the disease. But Hippocrates, as he himself said, considered the antecedent cause of the disease to be the plethos of blood, because the woman had not been cleansed by the so-called lochial purgation. The nourishment of the cause – that is, the genesis and first cause of the imperfect cleansing – was the distortion of the uterus, which was turned towards the hips.[28] So, since the retention was for him an indication for evacuation, while the tendency of the humours towards the uterus indicated the place through which the evacuation should be effected, he opened the vein alongside the ankle. Hippocrates is like that in everything.[29] But so that I may not annoy the Erasistrateans any more by praising him – for indeed it seems to me that they themselves, like Erasistratus before them, have it in for the man[30] – let us now leave the writings of Hippocrates; I shall have the opportunity at another

[27] K's text is corrupt, and the MSS are of no help. I render the probable sense.

[28] See K vii, 602–3.

[29] Caelius Aurelianus (*AD* iii.85) comments on Hippocrates' remark, which occurs in several places (L 4, 538; L 6, 134; L 7, 134) that cold water is beneficial in some patients, restoring heat; Caelius is surprised at Hippocrates for expressing such an opinion. Galen points out in his work *Causes of Symptoms*, however, that rigors may be due to hot rather than cold causes (K vii, 184, 190–1). Treating such patients with cold water does not contradict the rule of treatment by opposites; the cold water recalls the heat (K vii, 125–6). See also *De Temperamentis*, K i, 688–90. In his work *De Tremore* Galen says that rigor is due to the rushing out of the innate heat, which is obstructed and rebounds (K vii, 623). Asclepiades recommended bloodletting in tetanus, which some said was wrong, since the body needed the heat in the blood. According to Celsus, however (iv.6.1–2) it is not the nature of blood to be particularly warm. Galen would not have agreed; his point here, however, is that the patient, though shivering, was in fact hot.

[30] Galen frequently accuses Erasistratus of enmity towards Hippocrates, and at K 168 (see translation) says he holds his false opinions only because he will not admit to agreeing with him. Erasistratus, Galen says elsewhere, knew about the attractive faculty, but refused to mention it because he did not wish to refer to Hippocrates (K ii, 66). He would not admit that any of the humours was hot or cold, wet or dry, because of his feud with the school of Cos (K v, 685). Galen attributes the same motives to Praxagoras in his work on the opinions of Hippocrates and Plato (K v, 188–9); but there it is not Erasistratus who is in his bad books; Praxagoras' opinion on the origin of the nerves was so absurd, he says, that Erasistratus disdained to refute it! Galen's friends and enemies change places from one work to another; he is always polite to Hippocrates and almost always abusive to the Methodist sect, but all the others – even Plato and Aristotle – get it in the neck from time to time. It seems to be true, as Smith (1979, p. 198) remarks, that Erasistratus generally refrained from mentioning Hippocrates at all; it is thus impossible to know whether he was indeed hostile to him.

time to explain his whole practice where evacuations are concerned. Let us now pass on to the other men of both the empiricist and the K163 rationalist schools, for of these I do not find one who abjures venesection. Among the dogmatists, I know that Diocles, Pleistonicus, Dieuches, Menestheus, Praxagoras, Phylotimus, Herophilus and Asclepiades were phlebotomists, and this even although Asclepiades was so contentious that he overturned almost all the earlier doctrines, sparing none of his predecessors, not even Hippocrates; and not hesitating to describe the medical practice of the ancients as an exercise in death. But not even this man attained such a height of shamelessness as to dare to remove phlebotomy altogether from the list of medical remedies;[31] neither did anyone else, either of the present generation or of the ancients: not Mantias, not Athenaeus,[32] not Agathinus, not Archigenes, not the whole troop of the empiricists. Even among these men, who disregard theory and rely on experience alone, you could not mention a single one ⟨who held such an opinion⟩ if you looked at them closely.[33] What can be the reason why these men, who disagree on almost every other subject, have always been in agreement on this one? To me nothing seems more convincing than their universal lack of suspicion towards bloodletting. K164

But we will leave these men, if you wish, lest by the very profusion of witnesses we cast doubt on the works of nature which you praise. Does she not evacuate all women every month, by pouring forth the

---

[31] Empiricists trusted to experience alone; dogmatists had a theory (not the same for all of them) from which they derived their systems by logical reasoning. For an excellent account of the sects, somewhat before Galen's time, see Celsus, Prooem. 9–75. Galen has described them in his short work *On the Sects for Beginners* (K I, 64–105), the greater part of which is translated in A. J. Brock, *Greek medicine* (1929) pp. 130–51.

Of the physicians mentioned here, Diocles has already been referred to (see n. 7). Praxagoras is supposed to have discovered the importance of the pulse, unknown to the Hippocratic writers; he was both a pneumatist and a humoralist, and the teacher of Herophilus (3rd century BC) who extended his work on the pulse and the humours, and of Phylotimus (Fraser, vol. I, pp. 343–8, 355–6). Asclepiades (Rome, 1st century BC) is well known. Though Galen classified him as a dogmatist, he was not a Hippocratic humoralist; his system was materialistic, and everything depended on atoms and the passages they moved in. He rejected any idea of nature as a 'supernatural' power. He claimed to be able to cure safely, quickly and pleasantly, and was critical of the ancient physicians. Caelius gives a summary of his views (*AD* I.113–15) and says (*AD* I.119–23) that he used bloodletting only for pain, in which, he maintained, the larger atoms were involved; these could be drawn off only by letting blood. In phrenitis (frenzy), on the other hand, he regarded it as the equivalent of murder, since the small corpuscles were affected. According to Galen, who was prejudiced, Asclepiades had no regard for facts (K II, 52). For his life, see E. Rawson, 'The life and death of Asclepiades of Bithynia', *Class. Quart.* 32 (1982) 358–70.

[32] Athenaeus, who lived in Rome in the first century AD, was the founder of the pneumatist school, although the idea of pneuma and its connection with health and disease is of course much older. For Mantias see Fraser, vol. I, pp. 358–9.

[33] K's Greek is corrupt; I render what appears to be the sense.

superfluity of the blood? It is necessary, in my opinion, that the female sex, who stay indoors, neither engaging in strenuous labour nor exposing themselves to direct sunlight – both factors conducive to the development of plethos[34] – should have a natural remedy by which it is evacuated. This is one of the ways in which nature operates in these conditions; another is the cleansing that follows childbirth, although indeed the conceptus itself is also an evacuation, since it is nourished from the blood of the uterus; and the development of milk in the breasts after delivery is itself also an important factor in eliminating the plethos. The substance, after all, of the menstrual blood and of the milk is one and the same, one might say, and the veins are the common sources of the flow in both of them.[35] As a result, in those women who no longer menstruate because of their age, there is no accumulation of milk in the breasts either. And those women who are of an age to menstruate, but are lactating, have no periods. Further, if a nursing mother has a flow of blood from the uterus, her lactation is K165 suppressed. Among animals, those that do not become pregnant have no milk, and those that have milk are by nature subject to pregnancy. If you had the intelligence to understand further what great benefits accrue to the female sex as a result of this evacuation, and what harm they suffer if they are not cleansed, I don't know how you would be able to go on wasting time and not eliminate superfluous blood by every means at your disposal. A woman does not suffer from gout, says Hippocrates, unless her menses fail.[36] Yet why bother to quote Hippocrates to a man who is hostile to him? I see myself rather as a town crier shouting the truth at you, that a woman who is well cleansed is not seized with gouty or arthritic or pleuritic or peripneumonic diseases, and that neither epilepsy nor apoplexy nor suspension of breathing nor loss of speech occur at any time if she is properly cleansed. Has a woman ever been known to be stricken with phrenitis, or lethargy, or spasm, or tremor, or tetany, while her menstrual periods were coming? Or did you ever hear of a woman who suffered from melancholy or madness or haemoptysis or haematemesis, or

---

[34] For the accumulation of residues in sedentary women, see also Aristotle, *Gen. of An.* IV, VI.

[35] According to Aristotle, milk is concocted blood, and if a lactating woman conceives her milk dries up, since milk has the same nature as the menstrual fluid (*Gen. of An.* IV, VIII).

[36] L 4, 570. In Galen's commentary on the *Aphorisms* of Hippocrates, however, he says that women in his own time do suffer from gout while still menstruating; eunuchs get it too, although Hippocrates (same reference) says they do not. This, according to Galen, is because of the indolent and intemperate style of living in his time; in the austerer days of Hippocrates such people did not accumulate residues, in the absence of which gout cannot occur (K XVIIIa, 40–4).

headache, or suffocation from synanche,[37] or from any of the major and severe diseases, if her menstrual secretions were well estab- K166 lished?[38] And, on the other hand, if they are suppressed, she is certain to fall into every sort of illness. Thus even evacuations are healing remedies. But enough of women for the present; come now to consider the men, and learn how those who eliminate the excess through a haemorrhoid all pass their lives unaffected by diseases, while those in whom the evacuations have been restrained have fallen into the gravest illnesses. Will you not let blood from these men, even if they become synanchic or peripneumonic? Does your arrogance extend to letting so many die because you refuse to retract your mistaken notions? I would not put it past you; I, on the other hand, have often cured, not only these conditions, but even spasm and dropsy, by the removal of blood. This is what long experience has taught me,[39] and reason commands as well: to come to the cause and the nourishment[40] of the cause. You may confirm that experience also demands it, by reading the works of the empiricists.

6. Do not suppose, therefore, that your quarrel is with Hippocrates alone when he recommends the evacuation of blood, in cases where a man, through suppression of a haemorrhoid, or a woman, from K167 suppression of the menses, falls into a rigor, or a dropsy, or any other cold disease; you are at odds too with all physicians who rely on experience, and with the life of man, for you seem to me to be overturning the common doctrine of all of them. Would you not concede that the natural course anyone would take when faced with a plethos[41] of blood was to evacuate it? Who does not know that opposites are the cure for opposites? This is not the doctrine of Hippocrates[42] alone; it is the common belief of all men. You, however, because of your feud with Hippocrates, seem to have become more stupid even than irrational brutes[43] are. They do these things every day under the guidance of nature, curing hunger with feeding, and repletion with evacuation, cold with warming, and heat with cooling. What, after all, is the assimilation of nutriment but the establishment of a plethos? and what is defaecation but the evacuation of the

---

[37] Synanche or cynanche is an acute inflammatory condition of the neck and fauces.
[38] K does not have the question marks. The MSS never do, but Ju prints them.
[39] Reading ἥ τε for K's ἥτε. Galen was in his early thirties when he said this.
[40] K's ῥοπήν (so also Ald and Ch) is clearly a mistake for τροφήν, which, as already shown, was the reading in Galen's Hippocrates. A, U and M read τροφην.
[41] The Greek is corrupt. I delete διὰ and render the probable sense. A, U and M read σοι διὰ πληθος; A has a crux in the margin and an illegible word after πληθος.
[42] L 6, 52.
[43] Reading ἀλόγων for ἄλλων (conjecture of John Clement, *c.* 1540, pointed out by Dr Nutton).

overloaded bowel? What is micturition if not a cure for the full bladder? Those animals that feel the cold provide themselves with holes and warm burrows in the ground; those, on the other hand, that K168 are affected by heat swim in cold water in summertime, and spend their time in shady spots exposed to the wind. I have often seen the dog practising vomiting and the Egyptian bird[44] imitating the enema; men, who have the use of reason, are able to arrange all these things more skilfully than the animals can.

Call, then, a man with no medical training to a patient of good physique, young and full of blood, and suffocating from synanche or peripneumonia, and ask him if he has any views on the treatment; who would be so stupid as not to call for the evacuation of blood? But it is clear that Erasistratus, because of his enmity towards Hippocrates, does not share the opinions that are common to all the rest of humanity; he turns out to be even more unintelligent than the cranes. Even these birds can be seen from afar, like eagles flying to the ends of the earth, escaping heat and cold in turn, and curing opposites with their opposites in everything. As I have said, the idea that one should simply let blood from patients who are at risk of a plethos of it is not yet worthy of Hippocrates' art. I should prefer to have explained to K169 me the manner in which the evacuation should be effected, and on what occasion, and to what extent. To establish when one should cut the vein in the forehead, and when those at the corners of the eyes or under the tongue, the one known as the shoulder vein, or the one through the axilla, or the veins in the hams or alongside the ankle, concerning all of which Hippocrates taught[45] – this, I think, is the proper study of physicians. Merely to know that opposites are the treatment for opposites, and that evacuation is the opposite of plethos, does not impress me; even animals without reason have a share in such learning as that. But if you would undertake to open your ears, or, I should rather say, your mind, to receive the true doctrine, I might be prepared to overlook your hostility towards Hippocrates and tell you something worthy of that man's art. Even Diocles, Pleistonicus, and Herophilus, to say nothing of Praxagoras and Phylotimus and many other physicians, knew as much as this (not that they found it out for themselves; they followed Hippocrates): namely, when one ought to open each of the veins I have mentioned. K170 But how haemorrhoids protect against black bile is something not everybody knows, although in fact Hippocrates expounded it

---

[44] The ibis, which, according to one old author, 'purges itself at the fundament with its crooked beak'.
[45] The Hippocratic corpus, in fact, does not mention all these sites.

clearly.[46] Only those who apply themselves diligently to his works have learned from him how a haemorrhoid comes into existence,[47] and how dysentery, and how a varix; and how one should not always check these conditions when they have arisen, but rather learn on which occasions one should assist nature, and on which one should leave everything to her when she is untroubled in her action, and this is the proper course to take. So far are those who have this knowledge from hastening to cure dysentery, varices and haemorrhoids before the time is ripe, that they contrive to induce them artificially when they are not present at all.[48] For myself, I know of many patients who have lapsed into melancholy or gone mad in some other way when such evacuations have been checked through the ignorance of physicians. Some have been seized with pleurisy or nephritis; others have vomited blood from the stomach or coughed it up from the chest, or have perished from paralyses or dropsies. In my view the physician ought to know these things; it is an important branch of the Art that deals with evacuations.

7. How extensively one should evacuate when there is an excess of blood is not of great importance. Why ever, then, does Erasistratus fail to mention it, as one would expect of him if it were something of K171 significance?[49] And what nonsense are those people talking who are so ready to argue about everything, when they say that he did not know this about the evacuation, a claim they make in respect of other remedies too? For heaven's sake, what dosage do they suppose he could have calculated so precisely that he would never exceed the proper amount or fall short of it? For an enema, or one of the purgative drugs, or a diuretic, or food, or drink? Not one of them. The time has come for those who are constantly casting suspicion on everything to keep silence once and for all. Why ever did Erasistratus himself use purgative drugs, and give wine mixed with cold water both to cholerics and to patients with other conditions, assigning the credit,

---

[46] L 4 566. For the relationship between haemorrhoids and black bile, see K v, 117–18.

[47] For Hippocrates on the pathogenesis of haemorrhoids, see L 6, 436.

[48] A Hippocratic aphorism (L 4, 566) says that treatment of chronic haemorrhoids is likely to lead to phthisis or dropsy unless one pile is left untreated. Galen explains this in his commentary on the *Aphorisms*. Haemorrhoids, he says, develop when there is a plethos of thick blood, derived from the liver. If its escape is prevented by treatment of piles, the liver becomes cirrhotic, and its innate heat is extinguished, so that it can no longer generate useful blood; it produces instead a cold, watery humour, leading to hydrops. If, however, the liver is able to eject the plethos, sending it on to the lung, the likely result is the rupture of a vein, and phthisis. Hence the surgeon should always leave one pile intact, to excrete the faeculent cacochymia (K xviiia, 22).

[49] At the beginning of this work Galen accused Erasistratus of going into detail about minor matters while saying nothing at all about very important ones.

vulgarly enough, to his master Chrysippus for the discovery of a remedy known to none of his predecessors, and sufficient in itself for the cure of choleric patients already near to death? He did not, after all, administer it at any odd time, but reserved this remedy for very acute crises. I do not censure him for this as long as he could judge the proper occasions with accuracy; one may well wonder, however, at K172 the things he himself said, as if he were expounding some Chrysippean doctrine. Such was his boldness that nothing in the situation alarmed him: neither the acuteness of the crisis, nor the difficulty of determining the exact measure, nor the peril of the disease. No; he is convinced that he can clearly and at the same time precisely expound the exact measure and the occasion for its use, so much so that he considers his counsels useful, not only for physicians, but for laymen as well! Yet on those occasions when he ought to commend one of the ancients for his discovery, he evades the question altogether.

Come, then; I shall demonstrate this truth to them, that it is easier to find the proper measure in the case of phlebotomy than with any other remedy whatsoever. It is often possible to judge it from a change in colour, which may be of two kinds: sometimes from the actual colour of the blood as it flows, sometimes from the colour of the patient's complexion. Again, loss of consciousness marks, in all diseases, the limit of the evacuation, as does a slackening in the tone of the flow of blood, and an alteration in the pulse. The fact is that over this evacuation alone, and none of the others, the physician has complete power to stop it whenever he chooses. Whereas, on the other hand, if K173 you give a drug purging downwards, an emetic, or diuretic, or a cathartic for the chest or the head, the initial administration is under your control, but subsequent events are at the disposal of fate. There is great danger in the administration of purgative drugs, either of the catharsis not being set in motion, or of the concourse to the bowel not being readily excreted, or being excreted with distress, biting, colics and chills, or pulselessness and loss of consciousness, or of a grave disturbance of the entire body as a result of being evacuated either insufficiently or to excess. Indeed, the ultimate misfortune often ensues in this state; for the flow to the stomach cannot be stopped in the way you can immediately put an end to the bleeding by putting your finger on the divided vein. None the less, however, no physician abandons the administration of purgatives for fear of the effects that may ensue; after he has blundered once he merely takes care not to use them in that particular way again. But why pick out cathartics and spend time talking of strong purgatives, when mistakes in the quantity of any food do the greatest damage? How great this danger is, may be clearly seen in patients who, after being strongly purged, are weak K174 and in need of feeding up. In these, too great a reduction in diet enfeebles the faculties, while an excess, being a burden on nature rather than a source of nourishment, totally suffocates and extinguishes them. Should we then abandon the administration of food, because it is difficult to estimate the proper quantity? If so, you will have to give up practising medicine altogether, since you could not find any substance used in medicine that does not have to be given with attention to its proper quantity. You cannot blame phlebotomy alone in this. Mistaking the quantity, in either direction, does grave damage. Everyone agrees that excesses are most injurious; when the danger is small, however, there is no occasion to go to excess. Let, for argument's sake, a moderate evacuation be taken as three cotyles.[50] If you took four you would do the gravest harm, but two would be of some benefit while doing no damage at all, and you can always eliminate the extra cotyle with enemas, fasting, rubbing or sweats. Besides, there is nothing to stop you letting blood again if you wish to. But why am I saying so much in my campaign against ignorant men, who, in addition to talking nonsense about things that have no K175 rational basis, know nothing about the things they praise? They marvel at the utterances of Erasistratus and bestow the name of that man on themselves, calling themselves Erasistrateans; yet they know so little about them that they expound everything except Erasistratus' doctrine.[51] So concerning phlebotomy they utter such egregious and portentous absurdities as to make one stand amazed, not only at their lack of knowledge, but at their shamelessness as well. For although Erasistratus himself has clearly said, in his book on bringing up blood – the only book, in fact, in which he mentions phlebotomy – that Chrysippus used not to let blood so that the patient, who is perforce being subjected to starvation because of inflammation, might hold out, they say everything except this. Do you wish me, then, to pay attention to those people who talk nonsense on behalf of Erasistratus, when I have the very words of Erasistratus to consult? I would not think that this was a proper course for anyone to take. So let us hear his own words.

'Chrysippus,' he says, 'does far better, since he does not consider only the present, but takes impending dangers into account as well. K176 Bringing up blood is dangerous because the danger of inflammation

---

[50] About one and half Imperial pints, or 850 ml. A modern blood donor gives a maximum of one pint.

[51] This address converted the Erasistrateans, as the second work will show, so completely that Galen had to change his tactics; their last state was worse than their first.

is linked with it, and in the presence of inflammation the nutrition of the patient presents a problem; a patient who has been phlebotomised in addition to being kept long without food is in danger of fainting.'

He tells us clearly in this passage that he is aware of the risks of starvation; risks which, he thinks, must necessarily follow upon the rather long period during which, because of the inflammation, the patient is kept without food.

8. But I need not go back to the raving Erasistrateans to tell me why he said that food should not[52] be given to patients suffering from inflammation: I have Erasistratus himself expounding it, in the passages I quoted previously, both from the third book on fevers, where he deals with the inflammations that arise from plethos, and from the first book on injuries. In both these books he says, not once but many times, that the veins, when emptied by starvation, will be better adapted to receive back again into themselves the blood that has flowed out alongside. How does he put it?

'The practice of not giving food to wounded patients during the time when inflammation is occurring is also consistent with these principles; for the veins, when emptied of nutriment, will more readily K177   receive back the blood that has gone across to the arteries.'

Being an evacuant remedy, in other words, fasting puts an end to inflammations. He gives no other reason for using it in inflammatory conditions, than this: that the evacuated veins will more readily receive back the blood that has gone across to the arteries. Ye gods! Anyone who wants to empty the veins, then, must engage in a long struggle, when it is perfectly possible to achieve it without distress, and in a short time! I don't know how anyone could be caught tripping over his own feet more obviously than this. 'I do not open a vein', he says, 'so that the patient may be strong enough to bear the fasting imposed because of the inflammation.' But for the sake of what do you starve the patient with inflammation? 'So that I may empty the veins', he replies. Why then did you not empty them at the outset? I pity the man his errors. In addition to being at variance, not only with the manifest works of the Art, but also with his own doctrines, he turns out further to be ignorant of this question: for what purpose fasting is used. And this although Praxagoras, to say nothing of Hippocrates and Diocles, had already explained the use of it both adequately and K178 clearly; and he was not so simple as to suppose that fasting should be used to empty the veins, and that it was the only useful remedy for

---

[52] This negative is missing in K's Greek and in the MSS; the Latin translators of K and Ju insert it.

this purpose. So, by heaven, Erasistratus' search for an evacuant remedy leads him to the feeblest of them all, passing by the effective ones and those that are able to lead quickly to the effect he desires. But let that pass; let us grant that inflammations following trauma are to be treated in the same way as those due to plethos. How, then, are we to manage the same plethos when it persists in the veins and distends them? and when it extends into the arteries, how is it to be cured? My own view is that on all such occasions evacuation through a vein is the quickest way. Let the plethos be carried to the chest, and suppose that one of the veins in it is in danger of bursting; shall we not then perform venesection, but bind the limbs with wool instead? Will that be enough? For God's sake, if you are going to use a revulsive remedy, don't you know that phlebotomy is a far more effective means of revulsion than that? I have had many patients who were bleeding uncontrollably until, by opening a vein, I stanched the haemorrhage. But Erasistratus, it seems, is ignorant of this too; for it is not common knowledge which veins should be cut when particular parts are the K179 seats of haemorrhage.[53]

Since, therefore, venesection can achieve most effectively the results we now need to bring about, permitting as it does both evacuation and revulsion, what do you mean by wasting time as well as wasting your patient,[54] when it is possible to avoid both the actual rupture of the vessels and the consequent inflammation, and the restriction of diet that is used for the treatment of the inflammation? If the plethos is the cause of the rupture, then by emptying out the cause you will prevent the consequence; and if you prevent this, you prevent also the inflammation that results from the rupture; and if this is prevented, there is no longer any need for fasting. But you seem to me to be so keen to recommend fasting that you yourself are bringing about a condition that requires spare diet. What is so dreadful about a remedy that evacuates the troublesome material without itself causing any trouble at all?

9. But I am exhausting myself unnecessarily; let me remind you of your own words. Have you not taught us yourself, in your first book on health, where in explaining the origin of plethos in the veins you describe the remedies in order, and, while you regard the object of all of them as evacuation, you say nevertheless that different forms of evacuation suit different patients? As evacuants of the plethora, K180 however – for thus you see fit to call the plethos of nutriment in the

---

[53] Revulsion is effective only if the proper vein is opened; this is discussed in Chapters 7 and 8 below.

[54] A play on τρίβεις and ἐπιτρίβεις.

veins – you prescribe exercises, frequent baths, and light diet. You say that the same evacuant remedy is not suitable for all, because not all patients are accustomed to using all of them, some preferring baths, some exercises, and some vomits after dinner; and because not all patients are liable to the same diseases. One is subject to epilepsy, another to haemoptysis, and a third to diseases of the liver or spleen. We shall not, therefore, attempt to evacuate the epileptic with baths; you are quite right in laying down this principle.[55] Neither shall we prescribe gymnastics for the patient in whom there is any fear of a vessel in the chest bursting. For there is certainly a danger, in the violent exertions of gymnastics, that a rupture may occur in the chest of one who performs them, simply as a result of weakness, without any plethos being present. Teach us, then, how we are to treat him; for you too agree on the necessity for evacuation. We have the evacuant remedies of exercises and baths and light diet. But you yourself do not think it appropriate to use gymnastics. In the matter of baths you have said nothing at all; you have not told us whether we ought or ought

K181 not to use them for patients with such a condition. I shall set forth, however, what is plain, and has the sanction of experience; and if I may be allowed to play the soothsayer a little concerning you, perhaps even your opinion. You yourself, in your book on bringing up blood, make use of bandages and fasting, and revulse by these means some of the plethos; it is not appropriate to evacuate it with baths. I suppose that you would shun[56] the bath when a vein was already ruptured; and you have not said that you would wish to use it when there was a risk of one bursting. Even if you were not in fact of this opinion, the plain facts are enough for me. For the bath must do the greatest harm to all patients with haemorrhages, and the reason is clear, if it is true that the blood is rarefied and dissolved into vapours and spirits by the hot bath, so that it is incited to movement and raised up to form a swelling. Substances are rendered soft and weak by hot washes. How could they not readily suffer ill effects when they have become softer and at the same time the matter that ruptures them has acquired movement and swelling? Hence we shall not undertake to evacuate in

K182 baths those patients who are at risk of veins rupturing from a plethos of blood. So, as a last resort, we must have recourse to the third of the evacuant remedies, light diet. Come then; since you yourself make use of this in three ways, prescribing light diet, or scanty food that does

---

[55] K reads ὀρθῶς τοῦτο κελεύων, which I follow. U, however, has τουτο γε λεγων, and M τουτο λεγων; A is uncertain. An alternative rendering is thus 'As you say, making, for once, a correct observation.'

[56] Reading φεύγοντα with the Latin translators of K and Ju. K's Greek follows U and M.

not nourish, or no food at all, or ordering a vomit after dinner; let us see, then, how we shall manage a patient on a reduced diet. Shall we order a vomit after dinner? But we are wary about strenuous exertion in the gymnasia; should we not be equally so about using vomits boldly? Not even a layman would be ignorant of this. All that is left, then, is to prescribe fasting, or give scanty food of little nutritive value. Even though such diets do not nourish powerfully, however, they still nourish to some degree, and we do not wish to add anything at this time, but rather to take away. As a last resort, therefore, we shall use the laborious and exhausting measure, in truth like some sheet-anchor sufficient for every disease, of starving the patient to death. Will we be in any position then to jeer at Apollonius and Dexippus[57] for killing by starvation? I would like to remind you that you yourself have taught this doctrine, for you seem to me to feel as I do about fasting – that it is not an evacuant remedy. After I have demonstrated what I wish to K183 prove, I shall remind you of your own testimony. Fasting, I take it, is not one of the things that exist, any more than blindness or deafness is; rather all such conditions are deprivations of things that exist. The administration of food, however, is one of the entities that do exist, and as a result you can work out its function for yourself:[58] it is the nourishment of the body. Not giving food is not the same as one of the existing things; you cannot demonstrate any function for it, in the way in which you can assign an evacuatory function to sweats, phlebotomy and the enema, and a nourishing function to meals. Now fasting is midway between the two conditions, evacuation and nourishment; for it neither nourishes nor evacuates. How then is it, he says, that many people die of hunger for want of food? It is not for want of food, we shall reply, since if it were, it would not be possible for hibernating animals to survive while taking none. Yet they do survive, a fact that Erasistratus himself admits, and gives the reason.[59] Every

---

[57] Apollonius is presumably the one of Citium, who practised in Alexandria in the first century BC. See Fraser, vol. I, pp. 362–3. Dexippus may be the physician of Cos referred to in Anon. Lond. XII.8f.

[58] Reading αὐτός with A, U and M.

[59] The Anonymus Londinensis, the author of a papyrus incorporating the work of Menon, a pupil of Aristotle, describes an experiment in which a bird, kept in a pot with its excreta and presumably not fed, is found to weigh less after a time, showing that transpiration has occurred; the Erasistrateans, he says, maintain that this happens with man as well (Anon. Lond. XXXIII.44–53). Galen points out (K VIII, 281–2) that even hibernating animals have slight movements of the chest, and doubts therefore whether respiration through the surface of the body is sufficient for life; his point here, however, is that such respiration is reduced almost to nothing in hibernating animals, so that they do not require nourishment. Such contradictions are common in Galen's voluminous works. Galen says that respiration through the body surface is effected by the heart through the arteries (see above, p. 9), and that the same phenomenon occurs in hysterical women, who may appear to be dead; one

animal,[60] he says, naturally respires through its outer surface, either
K184 more or less, depending on its permeability. There are various factors
that increase or decrease the porosity of the surface, not the least
important of which are the changes in the body resulting from heat,
cold, inactivity and movement. When the surrounding air is warm and
the animal is active, the flow of material from it is greatest; when the
environment is cold, on the other hand, and the animal remains
motionless, the surface is thickened, and either nothing or a greatly
reduced amount flows away. For this reason, he says, hibernating
animals do not need nourishment. Seeing that their whole bodies have
become cold, sluggish and dense through inactivity, and the outer
surface is thickened in the cold of winter, which is the season when
animals hibernate, nothing flows away to the exterior, and as a result
they do not have to replace any loss. Nourishment has a function, and
animals put it to use to cure the lack resulting from evacuation.

It is clear, therefore, that the evacuation through the entire body
surface is the cause of the deficiency, and the function of food is to
K185 replace what has been eliminated. If the cause by which the animals
required food is abolished, it must be that every need for it is abolished
at the same time. This is why hibernating animals require no food; it is
because nothing needs to be added.

We have been shown clearly, then, that it is not the nature of fasting
to evacuate; it is the porosity of the skin that does it. And if you thicken
the skin with inactivity and cold, what further use is there for
starvation? Certainly we must beware both of exercise and of any
application of heat in the patient who is at risk of haemoptysis, since
exertion is liable to rupture veins by tension, while heating is dangerous for the same reason as baths are. If you do not heat, you will not
evacuate the body; and if you do, no matter whether you use exercises
or baths, you will do grave harm, by increasing[61] the tendency of the
veins to rupture.

What further advice, then, shall we give to those who are struggling
with this problem? Fasting, without exercising the patient or in some
way heating him, cannot evacuate; and phlebotomy, according to you,
we must utterly abjure, just as we must, I think, the strong purgatives.
K186 The abundance of evacuant remedies that can replace fasting is

Heraclides Ponticus reported such a case (K VIII, 414–6). Not only the postulated ends
of the arteries (see K II, 204–7) but those of the veins too were supposed to absorb
matter from the exterior. The Hippocratic work *Regimen* III recommends that after a
vomit the patient should gargle with astringent wine, in order to close the mouths of
the veins and prevent absorption of the vomitus (L 6, 608). See also Aristotle, *On
Respiration* VII.

60 Reading, with A, U and M, ἅπαν γὰρ φησι ζῶον κατα την . . .
61 Evidently a word has been lost here. The MSS do not provide it.

remarkable. If we are going to use it on its own we shall achieve nothing, since it does not evacuate by itself. And when it is used in combination with a natural evacuant, its deleterious side-effects outweigh the benefits of the evacuation.

CHAPTER 3

Galeni de Venae Sectione Adversus Erasistrateos Romae Degentes
Galen's Book on Venesection against the Erasistrateans in Rome

In this second book Galen explains the circumstances in which the first work was written and its effects on medicine in Rome when its contents were made public.

When I first came to Rome I found certain physicians who avoided phlebotomy so sedulously that sometimes even when a person was suffocating from plethos they refused to use the remedy. In the case of a woman almost twenty-one years old, who had a red face and a slight cough and already some difficulty in breathing, as a result of suppression of the menstrual catharsis, I found them lightly binding her limbs with woollen bandages and ordering her to fast, but neither using
K188 phlebotomy themselves nor permitting me to do so. Since they were more trusted than I was because of their intimacy with the woman's family and their seniority, I gave up for the time being the attempt to convince them concerning phlebotomy; I did, however, enquire whether there would be any objection to provoking a flow of blood to the uterus by means of drugs with the power to effect this.[1] When they agreed, I at once sought out the patient's usual midwife[2] and urged her to make use of them. She told me, however, that she had used them as the occasion demanded, when the monthly purgation was expected to occur, and mentioned the drugs she had applied to the woman; they were all of approved quality, so that no one could think the treatment had failed because of their weakness. Accordingly,

---

[1] These works give an interesting picture of medical practice and ethics in second-century Rome. Apparently, even if the patient was already under medical care, any doctor was free to offer his services and to prescribe treatment, as long as he was able to convince the family that he should. There is an amusing account in the *De Methodo Medendi* of a case in which the other doctors were unaware that Galen was also attending their patient between their visits, and countermanding their orders (K x, 536–42).

[2] This shows that the work of the midwife (μαιεύτρια) was not confined to obstetrics, but embraced gynaecology as well. For an earlier period, cf. Euripides, *Hippolytus* 293–4: 'If you are suffering from one of the ills that are not to be spoken of, there are women here, to help you set it to rights; but if your trouble may be divulged to men, speak, so that the matter may be revealed to the physicians.' In Aretaeus (IV.11.11) the prolapsed uterus 'readily goes back inside at the hands of the midwife'. Galen mentions vaginal examinations performed by the midwife at K VIII, 433–5.

when I had ascertained this, and also that the bleeding had now been suppressed for four months, I met with the doctors again and tried to persuade them to resort to phlebotomy. When they refused, I wondered whether they were planning to evacuate the excess of blood through the uterus, a thing they would obviously do by opening the veins that abound there, since they thought that if any other vein were K189 cut the evacuation would be harmful. When they replied, however, that it was possible to evacuate the excess of blood by fasting alone, without any such remedy being applied, I left them without further words, having lost all hope of a favourable outcome for the woman because of the cough and the dyspnoea. I expected her either to cough up some blood from the chest or lung, through the rupture of a vein, or, more probably, to develop synanche, pleurisy or peripneumonia.[3] I hoped, as a choice of evils, that the woman would become pleuritic, since I feared the acuteness of the danger in synanche or peripneumonia, and also the fatal effects of a vein in the lung bursting. This, in fact, was exactly what happened. With the increasing force of her coughing blood was being discharged upwards, and with a number of laymen already criticising the doctors who were preventing the woman from being bled, there was general hope that now at least, even if they had refused before, they would be shamed into consenting to the remedy. But when they did not yield even then, but ordered the bandages on the limbs to be tightened further, irritants to be K190 applied via the uterus, and the fasting to continue, I left them, having given up hope of achieving anything because of the seniority of the men and their reputation. The woman died soon afterwards in a fit of uncontrollable dyspnoea. There were some synanchic patients, who were prevented from being phlebotomised by these same doctors, who died quickly as well. Then there was another man, in springtime, who had been replete throughout the winter without exercise, and had his eyes and his whole face as red as someone's who had been leaning his head on the ground and stretching his legs upwards and continuing for some time in this position; on the fifth day this man

---

[3] For haemoptysis in women whose menses have been suppressed, see also Aretaeus II.2.9. The Hippocratic work *Prorrhetic II* says that the prognosis of phthisis in women is hopeless unless the menses are copious and regular (L 9, 24). The girl from Chios (see K 200ff. in the translation) was a patient in whom they were suppressed. Phthisis is distinguished from peripneumonia, an acute inflammation of the whole lung, by its long duration. If only a part of the lung is acutely inflamed, the condition is pleurisy (Caelius, *AD* II.141–2), which is less severe; hence Galen's hope that the woman would suffer nothing worse. The fluxion, however, need not settle in the lung; if it goes to the neck the result is the acute inflammatory condition of synanche, which may suffocate the patient. In the case of Criton (see K 208ff. in the translation) the inflammation started in the neck and later moved to the chest.

suffocated in an attack of dyspnoea. In addition to these patients, these enemies of phlebotomy were busy conducting to her death in the same way a fourth woman whose menstrual catharsis had been suppressed for a long time. They kept her without food, particularly for the first three days;[4] for, it is true, she had a continuous fever as well. On the fourth day they gave her a minute quantity of slops; then on the fifth day they again ordered fasting. At this point, in a violent
K191 paroxysm, she sprang up delirious and rushed out of doors shrieking, so that those present could hardly restrain her. Nature, however, saved this woman at least, by pouring out blood copiously from her nostrils. It was a source both of wonder and of edification to see how great a power the removal of blood has for the cure of such conditions; for immediately the haemorrhage from her nostrils occurred, the woman was relieved of all her symptoms.[5] Before this I had been afraid to argue with the doctors, as I guessed what they would say to avoid having to use phlebotomy. But now, since it seemed obvious to everyone that the woman had been saved at the moment when the evacuation of blood took place, I reminded them of those who had died, pointing out that if someone had phlebotomised them they might perhaps have been saved; and I mentioned some other arguments as well. But after twisting and turning my words upwards and downwards and getting nowhere, they finally took refuge in Erasistratus. In his first book on bringing up blood, they said, he had shown that binding the limbs was better then phlebotomy, while in his study
K192 on fevers he had made no mention whatever of venesection, as he would have done if he were referring to the things he had demonstrated in his book on bringing up blood. Indeed, they said, he would be ridiculous, if, having deprecated phlebotomy for the disease that seemed most to need it, he were still to speak about the others in this connection.[6] And they said that this same Erasistratus had been silent on phlebotomy, not only in his book on fevers, but also in all his other works. Neither in his book on diseases of the bowel nor in those on paralyses or on gout, nor even in his book on health, had he used phlebotomy, although in his writings on health he had admitted that a plethos of blood was a major cause of diseases. But when I expressed

---

[4] This is probably a reference to the celebrated diatriton, or three-day fast, prescribed by the Methodist sect for all feverish patients; perhaps the Erasistrateans also favoured it.

[5] Galen explains in his commentary on the Hippocratic work, *Regimen in Acute Diseases*, that in the acute fevers the material that has vaporised from the overheated blood is carried to the head (no doubt accounting for the delirium); when nature ruptures a vein in the nostrils and evacuates it, the disease is cured (K xv, 748).

[6] I.e. he said that phlebotomy was not necessary for haemoptysis, the condition generally thought to be the principal indication for it; he would naturally, therefore, not refer to other diseases.

surprise at their remarks and went on asking them whether phlebotomy should never be used, even when someone had peripneumonia or was suffocating from synanche, or when, through suppression of the menstrual purgation or of a haemorrhoid, the excess
of blood was driven into the chest, they replied to these questions by
citing the patients described by Erasistratus in his books on divisions,[7] K193
and of these particularly Criton and the girl from Chios. Erasistratus,
they said, did not phlebotomise the former, who was troubled with
synanche from the beginning and was at the same time plethoric, as
he himself wrote; nor the latter, in whom the menses were suppressed and the plethos was being driven into the lung. While they
were still saying this, however, a certain Teuthras, a fellow-citizen
and schoolfellow of mine – he was exceedingly frank in his ways –
said: 'You will never influence these men; they are too stupid to
remember the patients who were killed by Erasistratus. For what
other reason', he said, 'did the patients they are citing now come to
die, if not that the remedy of phlebotomy was omitted? And why else
did the patients die who were prevented by these men from being
evacuated in good time?' He enumerated them all in order, together
with the conditions they had, which I mentioned a little earlier; then
he smiled and threw up his hands,[8] and drawing me after him forcibly he led me away from the doctors. The next day he brought out
the books of Erasistratus on divisions and read them to all the philo- K194
sophers, with the aim both of showing that the girl from Chios and
Criton had died because of Erasistratus, and of trying to provoke the
senior physicians to debate; but they did not arrive, considering it
beneath their dignity to contend with a youth. At that time the
custom had somehow sprung up of speaking in public each day on
any questions that were put forward, and someone posed the question whether Erasistratus had been right in not using phlebotomy. I
dealt in detail with this question, which seemed a very good one to
those listening at the time; this was the reason why Teuthras also
urged me to dictate what I had said[9] to a boy whom he would send.
He said he was particularly anxious to have it since he was planning
to visit Ionia and was on the point of leaving. I was accordingly persuaded by my companion and dictated the speech. It so happened
that the book leaked out to many people; it was not deliberately

---

[7] The word (διαίρεσις) may mean divisions, distinctions, classifications, surgical
operations, wounds or dissections, but it seems unlikely from the passage referred to
that the subject was surgical; perhaps 'Classification of Diseases' was meant by the
title.
[8] Literally, 'moving back his hand'; some meaningful gesture is meant.
[9] Accepting Kotrc's (1970) emendation, με τὰ λελεγμένα.

spread abroad by him.[10] The work was composed in a manner not
K195 befitting a book but rather a lecture room, at the request of my friend
that it should be dictated just as it had been spoken. But even such as it
was, and having many deficiencies compared with the ideal, it
nevertheless seemed to achieve somewhat more than I expected. For
all those who now call themselves Erasistrateans have come round to
the opposite opinion, and are lining up all and sundry to be phlebotomised; not only patients like those mentioned earlier, but also those
who are in any way feverish. It seems, therefore, that some sort of
Stesichorean palinode[11] is called for, in which I shall exhort these men
to spend as much time as they like squabbling about words, but to
have mercy on their patients, and to abandon this violent habit of
attacking the other party. The fact is that one should not renounce
phlebotomy altogether; but then neither should one suppose that all
those whom Erasistratus would have ordered to fast require it, which
is what the Erasistrateans of today maintain.[12] It is not the easiest thing
to identify all who need the remedy, just as it is not easy to decide on
the amount to be taken, or which vein to cut, or the time to do it. I
think this is why Erasistratus himself omitted to mention phlebotomy
K196 in connection with any disease at all, thus clearly forbidding its use in
the one condition that most requires it. But surely, the Erasistrateans
say, in ordering fasting at the times when inflammation is actually
occurring, he wrote word for word as follows: 'For the veins, when
they have been emptied, more readily receive back the blood that has
gone across to the arteries, and when this happens the inflammation
will become less.' If, then, it is a fact that he recommends fasting as an
evacuant remedy, he will surely, they say, far more readily have
recourse to phlebotomy. Here, if what they are saying is that he
should rather make use of phlebotomy when he wishes to evacuate
quickly, they are talking excellent sense, except that in this too they are
neglecting the contra-indications that sometimes prohibit phlebotomy, which I shall mention in the course of my argument.

[10] This refers to the first work. It is not altogether clear whether Teuthras spread it
abroad or not; this is discussed below, p. 106, n. 42. Galen's works, however,
apparently had a habit of leaking out in this way. In his commentary on the
Hippocratic work *Nature of Man*, Galen says that he wrote *On the Elements according to
Hippocrates* at the request of a friend who was going on a journey, and it was spread
abroad, Galen doesn't know how. This was evidently not a bad thing, however,
since, he says, it was praised by all educated men, although a few ignorant ones
criticised it out of jealousy (K xv, 1–2).

[11] Stesichorus (sixth century BC) had to compose a palinode or recantation after writing
a poem in which he blamed Helen for the Trojan War. In his retraction he maintained
that she had never gone to Troy at all.

[12] Galen's first work has converted them completely; too completely, in fact. This is
discussed below in Chapter 5, pp. 102–4.

2. We must now enquire, not only what is best, but whether Erasistratus really did use the remedy. At the time when I first came to Rome, all the disciples of Erasistratus denied this; today, however, all the most celebrated ones I know of are of the opposite opinion, though they regard it as a minor issue. Hence, leaving out the others, I shall refer only to Straton, who was a constant associate of Erasistratus and K197 wrote from his house,[13] so that it was said of him that he was in the man's service. This man said that Erasistratus was deserving of praise because, among other reasons, he used to treat without phlebotomy diseases which the old physicians had tried to cure with it. And indeed it is clear from his own writings that Straton himself always undertook his treatments without phlebotomy. What wonder is it that Erasistratus follows Chrysippus the Cnidian in everything, when he has chosen in advance to abjure phlebotomy, just as that man did? So, it is clear, do Aristogenes and Medius, and all the others of Chrysippus' sect. As far as the welfare of their patients was concerned, therefore, it would have been better for those men to have believed that Erasistratus did use phlebotomy; for the Erasistrateans of today, however, it is better that they should not believe it. One would have to be quite mad to think that Erasistratus had been silent on the subject of phlebotomy in the diseases recently mentioned because he thought it right for the veins to be emptied and to establish this as the aim of treatment, if one K198 were arguing from the conditions[14] in which one found Erasistratus recommending fasting; yet this clearly must happen to those people who maintain that phlebotomy is a remedy equivalent to fasting. If, however, it is not equivalent, but there are differences, which the student may discover, so that it is sometimes better to make the evacuation by phlebotomy alone, sometimes by fasting only, and sometimes by both, then plainly the facts refute these people; for Erasistratus did describe those differences.[15] If, as they say, he did have opinions on phlebotomy, their theory contradicts itself either way. If it is equivalent, that is why Erasistratus neglected to write anything about phlebotomy, both in his study on fevers and in the other books I have recently mentioned. If, on the other hand, the

---

[13] Kotrc (1970) translates ἐπὶ τῆς οἰκίας αὐτοῦ 'in his house', and I render similarly, but Smith (1979, p. 194) on the analogy of a work by Bacchius entitled *Memoirs of Herophilus and his House* thinks that Straton was referring to a school of thought. Fraser (vol. I, pp. 357–8) suggests that Straton may have been an apprentice living in his master's household.

[14] Accepting Kotrc's (1970) reading εἴγε τις τούτοις πεισθείη. The whole passage, however, from 'One would have to be' to 'recently mentioned' makes little sense either in Kotrc's translation or mine, and the corruption probably goes deeper.

[15] Presumably when he said that starvation and bandaging were better than venesection (see above, pp. 15–16).

remedy of venesection is not in every way equivalent to that of fasting, they are not drawing the right conclusion in saying that we must provide evidence concerning his use of phlebotomy from what he wrote about fasting. And indeed here too their argument contradicts K199 itself, as it shows that fasting is useless. For even if it is true that an amelioration of the disease follows when the veins are emptied by fasting, we shall nevertheless omit[16] it, for this reason: that it is far better for those who have once evacuated the excess[17] to avoid fasting, which causes much distress to patients and brings sleeplessness and vexation, to say nothing of disturbances of the stomach and corruption of the humours in it, and sometimes even suppression of urine.

3. But that Erasistratus did not in fact use phlebotomy, is abundantly clear from the descriptions of patients in his books on divisions, in which he explains all the things that were done in the course of his treatment, and it is clear that he nowhere mentions phlebotomy. As it would be a major undertaking to quote them all, it will suffice to mention only those whom, as I said a little earlier, the old physicians had mentioned. One of them is described in the first book on divisions, another in the second. This would be an appropriate time to quote the actual words in which Erasistratus explains everything that K200 happened to the patients. In the first book, then, he wrote as follows:

'In the case of the girl from Chios, the first thing was that the occurrence of the menstrual evacuations was suppressed for a long time. Next followed a cough, productive of phlegm. In the course of time she started to bring up blood; this recurred during the time of the menstrual purgations, sometimes every fourth and sometimes every second month. And if, at any time on the days when the purgations were taking place, the ejection of blood also occurred, it coincided with them for three or four days, making it perfectly clear that she was now suffering from this elimination in place of the menstrual purgations. There was a concomitant fever on those days; then it remitted.'

Having said so much by way of preface, Erasistratus goes on to write about her treatment as follows:

'At first she tried treatment with potions, fomentations to the uterus, and pessaries, and the rest of the regimen adapted to this purpose, for there was, indeed, some slight thickening round the cervix uteri. When, however, the treatment not only proved totally unsuccessful, but during one particular menstrual period a heavy

---

[16] Kotrc (1970) reads παραληψόμεθα and translates 'if we are to employ fasting because a remission of the illness follows . . .'. I follow K and the MSS.
[17] Sc. by venesection, if my interpretation (see n. 16) is right.

feeling developed in the loins, though there was no discharge, while K201
the fevers were more continuous, penetrating somewhat into the
body,[18] and severe attacks of coughing followed, we therefore
abandoned the local treatment to the uterus. We supposed that it
would be difficult, while the fevers persisted, to bring on the
menses; we employed, however, the rest of the therapeutic
measures we were in the habit of applying in other such cases, and
in accordance with the usual treatment when expecting menstruation, we withdrew food.[19] The ejection of blood occurred only
once, and that for a short time.'
He has mentioned nothing more,[20] though we may suppose that pus
was also being brought up. There is no word of phlebotomy here,
although it would have been, to say the least, appropriate, as all
experienced practitioners know, to use phlebotomy as the first remedy
of all. Perhaps, however, one of those people who have no hesitation
in expressing opinions on any subject whatsoever will say that these
things were not done on the orders of Erasistratus as supervisor of the
treatment, though he lists them here for us so that none of the things
that were done should escape mention. A quotation, however, will
confute these people, where he says: 'We therefore abandoned the
local treatment to the uterus. We supposed that it would be difficult, K202
while the fevers persisted, to bring on the menses; we employed,
however, the rest of the therapeutic measures for other such cases,
and in accordance with the usual treatment when expecting menstruation, we withdrew food.' In these words Erasistratus shows clearly
that he is not merely describing the treatment given by others, but is
counting himself in and mentioning himself as joint agent in all the
things that were done in the case of the patient. For the words 'we
abandoned' and 'we supposed' and again 'we employed' and
'expecting', and in addition to these again 'we withdrew food', clearly
show one of two things: either that Erasistratus himself prescribed the
treatment, or that he agreed with the things that someone else was
doing. And indeed if he did approve of the things that were done, this
would be a clear indication of the opinion he had about phlebotomy.
Withdrawing food can mean one of two things, either taking it away
altogether, or reducing it; and Erasistratus says that this was exactly

---

[18] Reading, with La, ἦσαν, οἱ εἰς το σωμα τι ἐνεδιδουν; Kotrc (1970), 'litterae incertae'
may have had an unsatisfactory microfilm here. LSJ gives (pain) 'penetrates in-
wardly' with the authority of Aretaeus. Localised heats can spread in Galen's
pathology; see below, p. 73.
[19] Accepting Kotrc's (1973) emendations of ἐχρώμεθα ἢ for χρώμεθα ὡς, τἆλλα for τὰ τ'
ἄλλα, insertion of τὴν before περίοδον, and προλαμβάνοντες for προσλαμβάνοντες.
[20] Reading ἄλλο μέντοι οὐδὲν ἔφρασεν, ἀλλὰ ... Kotrc (1970) did the same.

what was done to the sick woman at the time when the periodic
catharsis was taking place. This agrees with all his other writings;
K203 nowhere was phlebotomy used, but fasting was recommended.
Perhaps, however, here too they will say that the woman was
phlebotomised, and that he omitted to mention the remedy in his
account because we are to understand that it was applied, even if he
did not say so. Why on earth, then, did he not keep silence about the
fasting too, since we might equally well understand that? And the
same goes for the potions and fomentations and pessaries also; if they
had not been described at all by Erasistratus,[21] we could, I suppose,
have understood that the whole lot of them were used by the
physicians. After all, the problem of understanding the things that
were done,[22] even if they were not described, is one that is common to
all the remedies. But Erasistratus set out to describe everything in
detail, in the interests of exact clarity, so that no one might have the
authority to add any remedies in the belief that they were applied to
the sick woman, or to take others away, in the belief that they were
omitted. Besides, his account is also in conflict with their opinion. For
if the woman really was phlebotomised, then fasting was employed
unnecessarily; or rather, if one must speak the truth, not only
K204 unnecessarily but also harmfully. I shall show this a little later; in the
meantime it suffices for the argument to say it was unnecessary. For
since at the time of the periodic purgations, when the excess was
carried to the chest, there was danger that the woman would cough up
some blood, Erasistratus, wishing to reduce the plethos, arrives at
fasting, which is clearly superfluous if he was using phlebotomy: a
remedy by which, in a moment of time, it would be very easy to
evacuate the superfluity of blood. The gynaecologists in Rome, at any
rate, were persuaded above all by their actual experience of events to
have recourse to phlebotomy at the time when the menstrual flow is
expected, and to prescribe neither rest nor fasting, but to give
melicratum in addition and large quantities of moistening food and to
allow the use of baths. After this it is the usual result – at any rate when
the women have been deprived of the proper amount of blood – for the
menstrual purgation to make its appearance, particularly when the
venesection is performed in the leg alongside the ankle. If, however, a
person using phlebotomy were to prescribe fasting in addition, not
only would he prevent ⟨the reappearance⟩ of the preceding menstrual
periods ⟨in patients in whom they had been suppressed⟩, but the

---

[21] Reading πρὸς ᾽Ερασιστράτου; so also Kotrc (1970).
[22] Reading, with La, ὡς το γε συνιεναι των πεπραγμενων. Kotrc has not commented on La
at this point.

catharses would also now be inhibited ⟨in women who hitherto⟩ had been properly cleansed ⟨by their menstrual purgations⟩.[23] For in K205 fasting the blood is dried up and becomes thicker, and hence is rendered less free-flowing. But if the patients bathe and take in addition some melicratum, followed by a meal, and drink some wine that is neither harsh nor thick, the menstrual purgations come on.

This, then, is why I said that fasting in addition to phlebotomy was used not only to no purpose but also even harmfully. And from the things that actually happened to the girl from Chios it is clear that phlebotomy was omitted. She spat some blood, which she would not have done had she been evacuated, and she died in an attack of dyspnoea, which would not have happened either. Phlebotomy has had its greatest test in our own time in Rome, through the great number of women who drink very cold water from snow, with the result that their menstrual purgations are either abolished or reduced;[24] but the doctors, by venesecting these women, keep them in good health, so that they neither spit blood nor are seized with pleurisy, peripneumonia or synanche. Hence they do not believe that the girl from Chios was venesected by Erasistratus; had this been done, he would not, in K206 his description of the other remedies, have neglected to mention phlebotomy as if it were one of slight importance, nor would he have made his evacuation by fasting[25] nor would the woman have died suffocating from plethos. But enough of her, for the present at least. Turning now to Criton, we shall add, in his own words, Erasistratus' account of what happened to the man. It reads as follows:

'Criton's illness began with plethora, for he fell into a synanchic repletion, or in other words an inflammation of the fauces and epiglottis. Those who fall into this condition usually suffocate and die in a short time unless they are promptly treated. Since Criton, then, 'is in this state, on the first day we treat him by heating him with sponges in the usual way as soon as we stop applying plasters,[26] so that he is continuously under treatment. He is also given small pills of castoreum to move his bowels, with satisfactory results.'

No one, I think, could fail to notice the attention with which he des-

---

[23] From 'after this' to 'deprived', and from 'If, however' to 'cleansed', the text is defective, and Kotrc (1970) does not translate. I render what appears to be the sense of the second passage, which is very obscure in K, with conjectural additions in brackets; the MSS are of no help.

[24] From 'Phlebotomy' to 'reduced' Kotrc (1970) declares the text defective; the meaning, however, is clear. It is uncertain whether drinking ice-water was a fad or the result of a severe winter; see below, p. 110. For the preparation and use of snow-water in Rome see K x, 467–8.

[25] Kotrc's ingenious emendation of ἐχεῖνος to ἐχένωσε must surely be right.

[26] Accepting Kotrc's (1970) emendation ἐπιτιθέμενοι.

K207 cribes all the things done to Criton. He mentions the vapour-bath with sponges and the use of plasters, and even the pills. Does he not make it clear how the patient was heated with sponges, and explain the other measures carefully in order? Yet he deliberately says nothing about phlebotomy, regarding it, apparently, as a remedy of the smallest importance. To me it is not appropriate to mention the minutest details in such accounts. But Erasistratus does it again a little further on, where he says: 'It seemed to me that the disease had undergone a metastasis,[27] and that the synanche had flowed down on to the lung and liver, with exacerbation of the fever.' He related that this translation of the disease occurred without distension in the hypochondrium. Here I think it is particularly important that you should apply your mind to considering what sort of meaning this account conveys to you, when he says that the disease had undergone a metastasis. Was it that the inflamed parts themselves moved across, or that the blood, the actual cause of the inflammation, flowed over? It seems to me that the first of the aforesaid things cannot be considered,

K208 but that the second is the truth. Sometimes I myself check[28] the plethos which has begun to attack a part, whereupon it moves over to another part because the first one has the strength to push it away. This seems to have happened to Criton too; yet for all that, Erasistratus never mentioned venesection. For what does he say? He poulticed the whole chest together with the hypochondria. But just as the metastasis of the blood that was in excess took place from the parts round the epiglottis and tonsils to the parts lower down, in the same way when it was ascending from the lower parts to the head an abatement of the fever took place, and a sign supervened showing that the origin of the nerves was affected. Listen again to this account of Erasistratus': 'When the patient was in the tenth day from the onset, and the sixth from the start of treatment, the fever came on very strongly, with some distortion of the neck, and later in the day some sensory loss developed, so that he was incontinent of urine,[29] and not long afterwards the fever abated.' Then he adds: 'Thus it seemed to me that

K209 the disease was undergoing a metastasis back to the head, and that during the metastasis itself the fever returned, and later increased further when the parts round the head became affected.' Let me now

---

[27] A metastasis is a movement of a fluxion from one part to another. It has been mentioned in Chapter 1 that accumulations of residues move about in this way if the excretory faculty in the part where they first settle is strong enough to eject them.

[28] Reading ἴσχω with La.

[29] Accepting Kotrc's (1970) emendation ἐκ ταυτομάτου προΐεσθαι. He (1973) reads La as 'ἐνερθέντο (ut videtur) προίοντο.' I think it reads ἐγερθέντος προιοντος, so that the meaning may be 'he passed urine when roused'.

say something to the man to counter this argument. You observe very correctly, O Erasistratus, that a metastasis of the disease took place to the head. But it would have been even better if you had not said 'of the disease', but rather 'of the cause of the disease', namely plethos. One would not say that the affected parts of the body themselves had undergone translation; in the same way one should not say that the disease did. It is better, I think, to say that the first disease ceased, and that another began again on the translation of the cause, which was, as he himself said at the beginning of the whole discussion, plethos. If he emptied this out, the cynanche[30] in the region of the epiglottis would not metastasise downwards from these parts, nor would it again be carried up from there to the head. Thus it is clear that Criton also, like the Chian girl, died through neglect of phlebotomy. It seems that even Erasistratus was aware of this; for what does he say? 'The cause of death seemed to be this: the matters carried to the lung.' It is a pity that K210 he was not in time to evacuate them, knowing as he did from the beginning that the patient had a plethoric tendency. If, then, anyone should choose to argue that it was unlikely that Erasistratus, being an excellent physician, and knowing that Criton had fallen ill as a result of plethora, and the girl from Chios through suppression of the menses, would deliberately have neglected to let blood, but that this man and this woman did in fact have blood removed, though he omitted any mention of it in his account – what then prevents me too from maintaining that any evacuant remedy I might like to mention was applied to the patients, but left out of the description? What doctor in his right mind would put up with me if I spoke in this way? And how did these deadly signs, originating from plethos, come to appear in them, and even death itself? They had no other cause than failure to evacuate the plethos. Who would tolerate it if we[31] were to say that the minutiae of treatment were described by Erasistratus, while phlebotomy and purgation with hellebore and scammony were left out, as being, for some reason, obvious to everyone? If, from the purely general statement that plethora requires evacuation, we are to K211 suppose that phlebotomy is indicated, since it is one of the evacuant remedies, why should not all the other evacuant procedures be mentioned as well? They must not say, then, that Erasistratus used only phlebotomy on his patients; they must add all the others as well –

---

[30] Kotrc (1970) reads κύων and translates 'paralysis'; this usage has the authority of LSJ. All the MSS have κιων, which can mean the uvula, but this could hardly metastasise. I translate 'cynanche', thus keeping the association with Kotrc's dog, without much confidence, since we know that this was what the patient had, and as a localised inflammation it could certainly move about in Galen's system.

[31] Accepting Kotrc's (1970) emendation (ἡμῶν for ἀνθρώπων).

enemas, emetics, purges, baths, exercises, rubbings, swingings, anointings, heating plasters – every single thing they use. It is not enough to say merely that the patient ought to be evacuated, and make an end of your account of the remedies with that; rather you must add, first, the mode of evacuation, and then mention the materials with which it may best be undertaken, and in addition to this the time and the amount and the way in which it is used; because, although he has mentioned the general aim of the remedies, he has not described them anywhere in individual detail. After all, if a general statement is all that is required, it is superfluous for him to mention the plasters and the fasting and the heating with sponges; we could perfectly well discover the plaster and the fasting for ourselves, without having to be told by Erasistratus. But phlebotomy, I suppose,

K212 is so obvious to everyone that Erasistratus does not even mention it.

4. This is clearly absurd; but even if one were to concede it to them, there would still be many other important questions to be considered by anyone who intends to use the remedy properly. First, whether it makes no difference which vein is opened, as some think, or whether there are special veins for each of the affected parts, which quickly empty out their plethos. Secondly there is the question whether it is appropriate to remove blood once or several times; and thirdly, of defining the aim of the treatment, so that the amount of the evacuation may be accurately assessed. The fourth question is at what time the venesection should preferably be performed, in the absence of any special contraindication. This will be explained, with proofs. For the man who abstains wholly from phlebotomy, there is no occasion to consider any of these matters; for anyone, however, who proposes to use it, it is obligatory to do so. And indeed the same argument applies to all the other remedies, such as hellebore, scammony, wine, bathing and foods. If none of the said remedies are used at all in the treatment

K213 of patients, neither the occasion nor the amount nor the manner of use nor anything else need be enquired into; but for one who gives his entire approval to their use it is necessary to go through all these things in detail. This applies not only to the most efficacious remedies, where if some small point is overlooked the greatest harm is done to patients, but also to the least. It can be seen happening any day with any patient. No doctor, for example, would say 'Let this patient be fed', and take his departure,[32] without adding the time at which he was ordering food to be given to the sick man, and defining the sort of food, the quantity and the manner of its preparation, and the arrangements for its use; no, he would explain all these things in detail to the

---

[32] Reading χωρίζεται with La.

attendants, saying how they ought to be done. What is more, in all their books doctors describe all these things systematically, in connection with whatever remedy they use; and some of them, by no means those most given to prolixity, spend time on these explanations, regarding such instruction not as long-windedness, but as solicitude. Hippocrates, who in most of his writings is brief in the last degree, none the less does not shrink from describing, in the matter of K214 phlebotomy, either the part of the body in which the vein should be cut, or the amount of the evacuation, or the occasion. Erasistratus, however – who, according to the modern Erasistrateans, used phlebotomy – although he is rather long-winded, as I shall show a little later, first of all could not find the time to write the one word, phlebotomy, alongside the other remedies; next, he omitted every one of the things I enumerated, the occasion and the amount and the situation of the vessel and the mode of use. And this from the man who did not shrink from writing about the necessity of applying plasters to each of his patients, or the mixing of barley-cake; who was not silent regarding the boiling of vegetables. Hear, for instance, what foods he describes in his book on the bowels:

'Give as the first course rough barley-meal, roasted and well shaken down. When you are going to administer it, give it after pouring water on it in some sort of wine-cooler, but not mixing all that you intend to give at once, but two or three times, so that the cake is neither hard to consume as a result of becoming dry, nor does it take up much of the moisture; for neither of these is beneficial. And you must also frequently give the patient to eat some chicory steeped in K215 mild vinegar; it should be eaten at mealtimes. Boiled chicory should be cooked by preparing two pots, and putting it into one of them to cook; when it is already properly cooked and the water in the other pot is boiling, transfer it to the other. There ought to be bindings so that the chicory is easily transferred. When it has been boiled and the water has been poured off, dress with salt and oil and give it to be eaten.'

Can you conceive it possible to describe the minutest details more carefully than this man does, who is not silent on the need to make bindings for the chicory, so that it is easily transferred? For the chicory, you see, becomes hard to transfer if it is loose, and so, out of solicitude not only for physicians like us, but also for cooks who boil vegetables, he has taught them that they ought to bind the vegetables together. He is like this too whenever he is describing the preparation of some plaster or other, or prescribing a walk of so many stades or a rubbing of so many rubs, or something else of the kind, so that already some people are not only denying him praise for his excessive attention to detail, but are even blaming him for his setting bounds and measures

K216 to things that are indefinite as to quantity. Who, then, could[33] be persuaded that such a meticulous person used phlebotomy as he did the other remedies, but did not mention it anywhere except once in his book on bringing up blood? And even there he was not using it himself, but, on the contrary, was praising Chrysippus for not using phlebotomy. There is also his account in which he expounds what he thinks was Chrysippus' doctrine concerning phlebotomy, saying that it is more generally applicable to those who spit blood than to all the other patients[34] in whom some part of the body is about to become inflamed. But more of this later. Now we must recall what I said, that Erasistratus, who protracts all his arguments to great length – and what is more, sometimes goes over the same matter in detail two or three times in different books – would surely not have omitted to put in, even if it was only once, five additional syllables alongside the other remedies, the word *phlebotomia*; nor would he further have neglected altogether to mention the quantity of it, as he does with the other remedies, and the occasion, as mentioned previously, and other such details.

Some physicians, at least, limit the amount of the evacuation by the
K217 signs, such as if there should be a change in the colour or the tone or the flow of the blood, or if the pulse should diminish in tone and sweating ensue during the removal of blood. They say that these are indications of distress, as are the most violent vomitings and unexpected diarrhoeas.[35] Others say that they continue the evacuation to loss of consciousness, as long as it is clear that this is due to the evacuation, and not to a humour flowing to the mouth of the stomach;[36] for it is often quite clear that fainting is due to bile or phlegm descending on it. Some decide on the proper amount to remove by the change in colour of the whole body, and by the pulse, and on these grounds they forbid[37] copious evacuation altogether; for they think it better that they should see what signs are yet to appear before completing in that way the evacuation of the troublesome matter. And some others have

---

[33] Accepting Kotrc's (1970) deletion of the negative in K.

[34] Kotrc regards the text from 'saying that' to 'all the other patients' as untranslatable. I render what may be the sense.

[35] Accepting Kotrc's (1970) emendations: ταῦτα δ' οὖν εἶναι πόνους φασὶν and ἄλλοι δ' εἰρήκασιν. He deletes the reference to Hippocrates and observes that the Greek is difficult to interpret. I render what seems to be the sense of the still unsatisfactory text.

[36] The cardiac orifice of the stomach is a very sensitive part in Galen's system.

[37] I follow Kotrc's (1970) emendation of ἢ χρῆσθαι to μὴ χρῆσθαι, but the passage (up to 'troublesome matter') is still obscure and the translation may not be correct.

been so rash as even to define some quantity, such as two Attic cotyles, as a moderate evacuation, or slightly more or less; so that, K218 using this as a mean, we shall be able to find out how much more or less will suit each patient who is phlebotomised, according to age, constitution, season and place. Is it likely, then, that Erasistratus would lay down some number of rubbings, even though no great harm would be done if we did not observe the exact figure, yet mention nothing at all in the matter of phlebotomy? I know well that he would have written a good deal about the particular veins that should be cut, and would have specially mentioned that Hippocrates had often referred to them, sometimes those in the ham or alongside the ankle, sometimes the straight vein in the forehead; or, again, the one in the tongue. And I need not add that Erasistratus would not have been silent concerning those at the elbow; he would have said either that one might cut any of them in any disease, or, as Hippocrates commanded, particular veins in particular diseases. It would be the natural act of one who describes everything so meticulously to set limits to any excess where such a powerful remedy was concerned, and to add his opinion on the veins, as other physicians have done. Some say that it makes no difference which vein one chooses to cut, K219 since the whole body can be evacuated equally well through any of them; others, however, take the contrary view that there is a very great difference, since some veins evacuate the affected part quickly, others in a longer time. But, as he neither writes anything about these, nor lays down the indications for the amount of the bloodletting, it is clear from his neglect of all these topics that he did not use phlebotomy at all. Just as someone who never uses poultices on patients cannot describe the different varieties, or their preparations, or the occasion or the way of using them, yet it is essential for those who do use them, as Erasistratus did, to pay attention to all these details, in the same way those who never use phlebotomy at all cannot describe the occasion and the mode of use and the principles by which the amount is determined. But for those who do use it, it is essential to distinguish all these matters, and particularly the differences between veins; if nothing else, at least whether it makes no difference to cut this one K220 rather than that, since all are equally able to empty the inflamed parts.

5. But not to write anything about these matters, and to make no mention whatever of any use of the remedy, and at that in the condition that has always been believed to need it most – how could anyone deny that this was a clear token of Erasistratus' never having used the remedy? When he wrote in his book on the treatment of fevers as follows: 'Round about the time, then, at which illnesses are

beginning and of the onset of inflammatory conditions, all sloppy food, in addition to solids, should be withdrawn', what difficulty would there have been in adding 'and phlebotomy should be used'? so that the whole passage would read:

'Round about the time, then, when illnesses are beginning and of the onset of inflammatory conditions, all sloppy food, in addition to solids, should be withdrawn, and phlebotomy should be used. For the inflammations that give rise to fevers arise for the most part as a result of plethora. So if nourishment is given at such times and

K221   digestion and distribution perform their functions, the vessels are filled with nutriment, and more powerful inflammations will ensue. It is better not to give food and to open a vein.'

His statement would have taken such a form if he had chosen to use phlebotomy also in the way he used fasting. Since, however, he has not made these additions, how could anyone believe that the man is praising the use of the remedy? And when it appears that he did not do this in any other work on treatment either, one may have further ground for confidence concerning his opinion. For who could believe that the very long-winded Erasistratus would shrink from adding, even if only once, a further four or five syllables to the bulk of his written works? For myself, then, even if no book of Erasistratus' had survived, but they had all perished already, as is in danger of happening to the works of Chrysippus – I would rather trust his disciples when they spoke of their master than people who had never seen Erasistratus himself, nor a disciple of his, or of any of his fellow-students, or of those who had been their associates. Yet after so

K222   many ages they boldly pronounce on things that they have never seen, nor heard from anyone who had seen, nor read, even if it was only four or five syllables, as I said, in the works of Erasistratus. For the words 'to cut a vein' consist of four syllables; *phlebotomia* itself is five. And the addition I made to his account a little earlier, 'one should make use of phlebotomy' is pronounced with nine syllables. So now let them desist who are doing damage, not only to those who are learning the art but also to the sick themselves, by saying that Erasistratus did use phlebotomy, but made no mention of it because it was more obvious to everyone than the boiling of plasters and vegetables.[38] If those who are learning the art are going to use phlebotomy because the venesections dissolve the inflammation in

---

[38] Kotrc (1970), whom I do not follow, emends the text to mean 'the use of plasters and the boiling of vegetables'. But Galen has Erasistratus boiling plasters and vegetables again in the first bloodletting work (see translation, K 147); Aretaeus boiled plasters (v.10.10), and so did my own mother.

exactly the same way as the emptied veins do in fasting, then they will phlebotomise every single one of those patients for whom Erasistratus ordered fasting. This, however, is an unimportant matter.

6. But the fact that the new physicians have recourse to the remedy without knowing anything about the amount of blood that should be K223 let and the veins that should be cut will do the greatest harm to patients, as I said right at the beginning. It would be better for them to renounce phlebotomy altogether than to use the remedy without paying attention to such matters. More patients have been lost in this way in the past than have died at the hands of those who did not use phlebotomy. The old practitioners of those days, who never used phlebotomy at all, employed other evacuant remedies which could achieve, although in a longer time, the same effect as phlebotomy, except where, because of the vital nature of the affected part or the excess of the plethos, the patient forestalled them by expiring. Today's doctors, however, who think that every onset of fever demands phlebotomy,[39] do no inconsiderable harm to the sick. For they have persuaded themselves concerning the remedy, just as if Erasistratus had actually written in the way I mentioned a little earlier, when I inserted nine syllables into his account to give a reading like this, for it is better to quote it from the beginning: 'Round about the beginnings of diseases and the onset of inflammation one should withdraw all sloppy foods as well as solids, and phlebotomy should be used.' This K224 is what the men of today would like Erasistratus' opinion to have been, but it is not for the good of patients, since there are some occasions when fasting is indicated, and others that require phlebotomy. I shall expound them in this work in due course. But now, just as they, who had previously accepted the views of the old physicians, have begun a new[40] recantation, so I too ought to make my palinode and bring those who are now phlebotomising irrationally round to not phlebotomising at all. For as Plato said, people who do not so much as attempt things they do not understand are less likely to fail than those who undertake projects about which they are ignorant. This is what the men of today do, having misled themselves. It is, after all, easy to find out, first those whom it is necessary to phlebotomise, and then each of the other matters I spoke of. But they use phlebotomy in exactly the same way as they use fasting in the early stages of every disease. In fact, to tell the truth, they have changed the doctrine of Erasistratus; for they phlebotomise and then feed the patient forth-

---

[39] In his work *Against Julian* Galen describes the followers of Thessalus, who phlebotomise all feverish patients, as a herd of donkeys (K XVIIIa, 274).
[40] Reading καινῆς with K's Latin translator.

with, whereas he forbade phlebotomy and recommended that food
K225 should not be given. Since, therefore, these people do not honour the
truth but Erasistratus,[41] it is necessary to show them that the account
he wrote in his book on bringing up blood does not apply only to this
condition, but to all inflammatory diseases. His account, then, reads
as follows: 'For the danger of bringing up blood is associated with the
danger of inflammation, and in the presence of inflammation the
nutrition of the patient presents a problem; a patient who has been
phlebotomised in addition to being kept long without food is in
danger of fainting.' Such is his account of those who spit blood. He
forbids phlebotomy in these patients because he fears that inflammation may supervene, in which event, he says, it is not easy to
nourish the patient, or in other words to give him food; and that the
patient who has been phlebotomised and is also kept for a long time
without food is in danger of his strength failing. What he says here
does not apply only to bringing up blood; both parts of it are equally
applicable to fevers, the necessity not to give food because of inflammation, and the fact that if this is done to a phlebotomised patient
there is a danger of his strength being dissolved. And if you consider
K226 the matter carefully you will come to see that the said argument of
Erasistratus forbids phlebotomy in feverish patients even more than in
those who spit blood. In the early stages of bringing up blood the
ruptured vessel is not at all inflamed; yet the origins of fevers,
according to Erasistratus, necessarily involve the beginning of
inflammation.[42] If indeed, then, as that man himself wishes, we are to
use things that are clearly apparent to establish our belief about those
that are not clear, look at all those wounds that have forestalled us by
uniting before the patient has been phlebotomised. Hence it is
possible that the ruptured vein also need undergo no inflammation at
all, if we catch it in time by taking the other appropriate measures, and
by letting out some of the blood that is about to cause inflammation, to
whatever extent we think proper. If indeed then Erasistratus says that
in the time when the affected parts are becoming inflamed it is
essential to use fasting, and in view of this to avoid breaking down the
patient's strength in advance by phlebotomy, we ought to be far more

---

[41] Accepting Kotrc's emendation of οὗτοι τιμῶσιν, οὐκ Ἐρασίστρατον to οὐ τιμῶσιν ἀλλ'
Ἐρασίστρατον.

[42] This is Erasistratus' famous doctrine that fever is always the result of inflammation.
Celsus (III.10.2–3) says that he was greatly in error in believing this, and Soranus, as
echoed by Caelius, also denied it; some fevers, he says, come from looseness (*solutio*).
(This is Methodist doctrine, according to which all diseases are due either to
constriction or to relaxation, or a mixture of the two.) Besides, fever is not a necessary
sign of a dangerous disease (Soranus implies that Erasistratus said it was) since
patients with cholera are afebrile (*AD* II.178).

cautious in using it in feverish patients than in those who are bringing up blood. For in those patients it is possible for the ruptured vein to heal without becoming inflamed, particularly when they have been K227 evacuated; but in feverish patients the part must of necessity already be inflamed. One can believe that it is possible for the vein to unite without becoming inflamed from what can happen in all other wounds. I have often seen among the gladiators a whole leg or arm that has been cut open heal without becoming inflamed, and particularly when, as Hippocrates said,[43] an abundant flow of blood had immediately taken place. I have also often seen a puncture in the so-called empty part of the chest heal by the third day. Recently, too, a man who had received a blow in the wrestling school immediately brought up, in a violent fit of coughing, about two cotyles of blood; but after being bled at once and the other necessary things done, he did not cough again and remains in good health. From these examples I think one can see that in the case of those who have already begun to suffer from inflammation one ought to abstain from phlebotomy, if Erasistratus is to be believed, more rigidly than in the case of those K228 who have as yet no inflammation.

7. It is also no less clear than this that Erasistratus did not use phlebotomy, either in combination with fasting or instead of it.[44] Nevertheless, some have come to such a pitch of contentiousness and stupidity that when they hear such doctrines they make no attempt to solve the problem, but as if nothing had been said they start their own argument by quoting that one passage in which Erasistratus says 'It follows that no food should be given at the times when inflammation is occurring; for the veins, when emptied, more readily receive back the blood that has gone across to the arteries, and when this happens the inflammation will be diminished.' Then, on this basis, they say that the use of phlebotomy is clear. For surely, they say, wherever he makes specific use of fasting as an evacuant remedy, he will far more readily have recourse to phlebotomy. If someone should allege in reply that they have not proved by what they say that Erasistratus used phlebotomy, but that what follows from his remarks on starvation is that he did not use phlebotomy,[45] they laugh and say 'So you K229 can see what follows, I suppose, but Erasistratus could not? He must

---

43 Perhaps L 5, 236. See also K x, 378 for healing without inflammation. For an interesting account of Galen's gladiatorial experience, see J. Scarborough, 'Galen and the gladiators', Episteme 5 (1971) 98–111.

44 Reading προ αὐτων with La and K's Latin translator.

45 Accepting Kotrc's (1970) emendations: οὐ τομίαν to οὐ παραλαμβάνειν φλεβοτομίαν, τῆς εἰρημένης to τοῖς εἰρημένοις, and τῷ καὶ τῇ φλεβοτομίᾳ to τὸ μὴ τῇ φλεβοτομίᾳ.

have been unskilled in logic, which you have had more training in than he had, and if he were alive we would have advised him to become your pupil, so that he might get some practice in knowing what follows and what is contradictory.' Then they start offensively insulting those they are arguing with, stringing together abuses in such quantity one after the other that no one can get a word in, and that, as far as they are concerned, is the end of the discussion. We, however, are not looking for repartees to use when people start vilifying us, but for the answers to two questions: first, whether Erasistratus used phlebotomy, and secondly the question of the efficacy of the remedy. Each of these has its own proof. The proof that the man did not use phlebotomy is in his own writings and those of his most trustworthy disciples, and in the whole doctrine of Chrysippus;

K230 these do not apply to the question of efficacy of remedies, but here there are certain true premises together with the conclusions appropriate to them. If, however, anyone chooses to neglect all these, because his only wish is that consistency be encouraged, he will be in danger of believing that the things that were clearly written by Erasistratus were not written at all. Let us begin, then, by considering the exact words that Erasistratus himself wrote in his book on bringing up blood, where he is praising Chrysippus for rightly using bandages to the limbs in place of phlebotomy:

> 'This is the same effect that the phlebotomists wish to achieve in patients who bring up blood. Chrysippus, however, is far better, since he does not consider only the present, but takes impending dangers into account as well. Bringing up blood is dangerous because the danger of inflammation is linked with it, and in the presence of inflammation the nutrition of the patient presents a problem; a patient who is phlebotomised in addition to being kept long without food is in danger of fainting.'

He has not added the reason why he thinks it right to use starvation at the time when inflammation is occurring, since he has spoken of that

K231 in another passage in which he says:

> 'The practice of not giving food to wounded patients, during the time when inflammation is occurring, is also consistent with these principles; for the veins, when emptied of nutriment, will more readily receive back the blood that has gone across to the arteries, and when this happens the inflammation will become less.'

Thus he approves of fasting when inflammation is occurring, because it empties the veins. But if you combine the two passages quoted, the result will be something like this: 'Chrysippus was right in not phlebotomising patients who bring up blood, because a little later they

will need the evacuant remedy of fasting.' And the same argument
again, if expressed more briefly, would be something like this: 'One
ought therefore not to evacuate patients who are bringing up blood,
because soon afterwards, when inflammation is occurring, they will
need evacuation.' Or it might be put even more clearly as follows:
'Before the time of inflammation one ought not to evacuate the veins,
because when they are emptied the inflammatory condition is
checked.' It is quite clear that the argument contradicts itself, unless
anyone should rashly try to defend it by maintaining these two K232
propositions: that it is better to evacuate the body at the actual time of
inflammation rather than before it has started, and that fasting is
preferable to phlebotomy. If these provisos are not made, we may say
that the proposition has not been proved, neither is it self-consistent;
for the parts of the argument are dissimilar and logical order is not
preserved. It is clear, after all, to anyone who has even a particle of
sense that for one who has made it his aim to bring back to its proper
place, by emptying the veins, the blood that has gone across to the
arteries, this should be done as quickly as possible.[46] It is clear also that
one should use an evacuant remedy that is able to effect the evacuation
in the shortest possible time, and without doing harm to the body. It
has been shown a little earlier what grave damage fasting often does to
the sick. One might say, therefore,

'I think those people who suppose that Erasistratus used venesection on patients who bring up blood are quite ridiculous. For
where he recommends fasting as an evacuant remedy, he must
surely be recommending it in preference to phlebotomy. And since K233
he thinks it necessary to go on evacuating during the period in
which inflammation is occurring, it is clear that he will also recommend evacuation when the inflammation is beginning or is about to
begin. Erasistratus, after all, was intelligent enough to realise that he
could transfer the blood much more promptly back from the arteries
to the veins at the beginning of its passage across, when it had not
yet become tightly packed in, or dried up by the feverish heat which
had thickened it.'[47]

Anyone who maintains that this is not so is clearly showing himself to
be ridiculous, not those whom he is accusing; since Erasistratus
himself has written that he did not use phlebotomy, thinking it better
to avoid its use when inflammation is taking place.

---

[46] Accepting Kotrc's (1973) emendations: ἐναργὲς for ἐναργῶς, ὁσοιπερ for ὁσοι γὰρ,
and ὡς τῷ σκοπὸν ὑποθεμένῳ for ὥστε σκοπεῖν ὡς θεμένῳ.
[47] Accepting Kotrc's emendations. He inserts ὡς ἀγνοεῖν before ὅτι θᾶττον, and
emends οὔτε σφηνούμενον to οὔτ' ἐσφηνωμένον.

8. To keep in check what is incurable, or what is difficult to cure, such as also follow haemorrhoids.[48] When we said that the bandages on the limbs were sufficient to bring the plethos to themselves without phlebotomy, he[49] replied that this was impossible in plethora, in K234 which condition Erasistratus had himself said that the arms, hands and lower legs were inflamed, as a result, according to him, of the plethos of blood distending the vessels. How then could the material in the deep parts move across to them, when it is clear that even without it they are already in danger of bursting? And indeed, I said, Erasistratus praised Chrysippus, not by analysing his argument, as I shall now do in this account, but simply by stating it. The passage is as follows: 'Woollen bandages should be applied at the armpits and groins.' He says that bandages should be applied, without adding any further particulars as to whether the procedure will be ineffective in plethoric patients but beneficial to the others; he simply states it, so that we may see that it applies to all patients. 'He did not', he said, 'add "in all cases", by writing something like this: "to apply woollen bandages in all cases", but simply said "to bind with woollen bandages both at the armpits and at the groins", as if we could know that K235 the statement applied to those in whom it is possible to transfer some of the blood to the limbs; since in those patients in whom it is impossible there is no occasion to undertake treatment with bandages to the limbs.' 'Why ever then,', I said, 'did Erasistratus not write exactly what you have just said: that in those who are plethoric in this way, in whom the upper arms, legs and forearms are inflamed, it is proper to remove blood, but to bandage the limbs in the others?' 'Because', he said, 'he was writing for people of more than ordinary ability to draw conclusions and to put them into practice, who would not attempt things that were totally impossible.' 'You are ordering us, then,' I said, 'not to bandage, whenever there is a plethoric condition in the body, even if Erasistratus did not mention phlebotomy in his writings, obviously because it was plain to all and so it was unnecessary for him to refer to it. He did, however, describe the treatment of the other diseases that are not associated with plethora.' When he had agreed with this, I asked him to listen first to a passage from the third book on fevers, and then to one from the first book on health. The third book on fevers tells us:

K236   'Round about the time, then, at which illnesses are beginning and of

---

[48] A most obscure remark; perhaps some reader's note that has got into the text. But the text, as Kotrc (1970) rightly observes, is incomplete here.

[49] It is not clear who this 'he' is; he seems to be an Erasistratean opponent with whom Galen is arguing, and the passage in which he was introduced has been lost.

the onset of inflammatory conditions, all sloppy foods should be withdrawn together with solids, for the inflammations that give rise to fevers arise for the most part as a result of plethora. So if nourishment is given at such times and digestion and distribution perform their functions, the vessels are filled with nutriment, and more powerful inflammations will ensue.'

In this passage Erasistratus clearly wrote the word plethora, and in expounding its treatment he mentioned fasting, but said nothing about phlebotomy. So I said to the Erasistratean: 'My good sir, you are wrong four times over, since it is clear that Erasistratus did write about the treatment of plethora.' And so again in the first book on health: after describing the signs of plethora by way of preface, he lists the remedies in order, and includes everything except phlebotomy. The passage is as follows:

'There is need for people to keep the closest watch on their health, by knowing in advance how to recognise and to guard against the K237 condition of plethora. Hence, for preference, one ought to dissolve it, not once it has actually started, but rather when it is approaching, before the illness has begun.[50] There are many ways of dissolving such a condition, and they do not all suit everyone; hence they will be discussed in order. For those who are in the habit of exercising their bodies the most effective method would be to do a little more of the customary exercises, to try to break up the abnormal condition, and after the exercise to be sweated in the bath, or to be dried out with hot applications in the usual manner, or to use the bath more freely, and after all these to rest and take no food for a longer time than usual; for this time after the exercises and the bath is particularly effective in destroying the plethora if the patient takes more rest and abstains from eating. In the succeeding period breakfast should be eliminated and the patient should take a smaller dinner, while the amount of food that he does take should be of a less nourishing kind. There should be various vegetables, raw and K238 boiled, gourds and cooked figs as well as the soft variety, green figs and a little pulse cooked with vegetables, and bread not of the fancy kind, since all these things make the bowels excrete freely, while the nourishment distributed from them is neither abundant nor strong. The patient should abstain, during the period in question, from meat, fish, dishes cooked with milk, unground salt and all such things, or use them much more sparingly. One must use this system of treatment so that the plethora which has collected may be safely

---

[50] From 'There is need . . .' to 'has begun' the text is unsatisfactory, and the meaning is not clear. I render the likely sense.

purged. For those whose bodies are not accustomed to exercise, it is inappropriate to impose more gymnastics, since at the beginning of the illness there may be fatigue in addition to the pre-existing condition, but rather to treat with sweating, bathing and fasting;[51] these effect safe evacuations for most people alike. It is generally useful, in all who vomit easily, to provoke vomiting after dinner, unless they are unsuited to it for some other reason, not leaving much time after the meal, so that the vomit catches the food higher

K239   up[52] and there is not much distribution of it beforehand. The next day the patient should take breakfast and have baths and sweats. When the body has been evacuated and recovery from the plethora has taken place, he should soon return to his accustomed way of life.'

In this account Erasistratus has explained everything clearly. He himself uses the other remedies in the plethoric diathesis, but he does not use phlebotomy. He implies this again further on in his account, where he says:

'It is also necessary to understand these matters because not all people suffer from this disease in the same way. Although the same signs – I mean plethora – develop in many people, the part attacked is not the same in all; in some it is the liver, in some the bowel, in some an epileptic condition results, and in others the joints are affected. It is necessary, therefore, to consider what is usual for each patient and take the precautions appropriate for the diseases that are developing.[53] One must not take the same precautions for a

K240   patient who is liable to epilepsy as for one who is given to haemoptysis; for the former one should prescribe strenuous exertion, but tiring exercises must be avoided for the latter, since rupture may be initiated by exertion. In the same way a patient subject to epilepsy should be given over to unremitting fasts and restricted diet, while frequent baths and anything causing violent change must be avoided. One suffering from kidney disease should take a light diet and use the bath liberally; his drinking should not be reduced, so that his urine does not become acrid and ulcerate the

---

51 La has a passage, not in Kühn in either Greek or Latin (from 'since at the beginning' to 'sweating, bathing and fasting') which has been pointed out by Kotrc (1977). It reads, according to him (either my microfilm was less legible or Kotrc was more accomplished): μήποτε κόπου προσγενομένου τῇ προϋπαρχούσῃ διαθέσει ἀρχὴ ἀρρωστίας γίγνηται, ἀλλ' ἱδρωτοποιίας τε καὶ λουτρὰ καὶ ἀσιτίας ἐμβάλλειν.

52 Reading, with La, ἵνα μετέωρα τε τα σιτια λαμβανεται προς το ἐμειν. I think the meaning is that the artificially provoked vomit intercepts the food before it has been able to descend far.

53 Accepting Kotrc's (1973) emendation. He reads συννοοῦντα τὰ εἰθισμένα for συνθρωτὰ εἰθισμένα.

passages through which the excretion is conveyed. Vigorous exertion is irksome to these patients. For those who are subject to diseases of the spleen or liver one must beware of fatigue and cold baths, and must generally take precautions by using fasting, restriction of drink, and baths.'

9. In this passage Erasistratus has again clearly shown what his opinion is. Those who, as a result of plethora, are at risk either of haemoptysis or of epileptic seizures, he makes no attempt to evacuate K241 with strong purgatives, nor with frequent rubbing, a remedy weaker than this although considerably stronger than fasting by itself; so much so, in fact, that with it I have evacuated some patients who were too faint-hearted to take a purgative or allow a vein to be opened. If this remedy were sufficient in all cases, perhaps it could be used routinely in place of phlebotomy. In fact, however, it is sometimes found more irksome than the plethora that is affecting the body, particularly by those who are unaccustomed to massage, who are overcome with fatigue at once if they are thoroughly rubbed. Others, again, have thick hard skins, and even if thorough rubbing is applied, only a very brief evacuation results. Any doctor who diligently studies the operations of the Art, with experience herself as his teacher, will know that emptiness of the stomach invites an epileptic fit. He will know of patients who are seized with epilepsy upon a mere disturbance of the stomach, some of whom are greatly harmed by fasting, as K242 was Diodorus the grammarian. This man, if he ever went long without food when producing some literary work, had an epileptic seizure. As a remedy for him I arranged that he should take some bread dipped in diluted wine at the third or fourth hour, and with this treatment he has remained in good health for many years through paying attention to only one thing, the best possible digestion of the food after the meal. And when, because of some business of state, he had to spend the time till noon in the forum without eating, he fell down in a convulsion. This man, as I said, was seized with epilepsy when his stomach was disordered. For the injured stomach clearly incites the other organs to convulsions and quickly draws them along with it, whenever it is appropriate to do so, even if it does not happen always. Sometimes the mouth of the belly is called the stomach by doctors when speaking of such conditions.[54] Many of my predecessors have

---

[54] For another patient like Diodorus, see K viii, 340–1. From 'For the injured' to 'such conditions' the text is defective, and I render what seems to be the sense. The sentence about the mouth of the stomach frequently occurs in Galen; it is probably a gloss here. The mouth of the belly, or cardiac orifice of the stomach, is the sympathetic organ par excellence; what happens to it affects other parts of the body, and vice versa. This is because it is joined by one of the most important nerves from

been aware of conditions like this, but it would be better to speak of
K243 them elsewhere. In the present work I shall go only so far as to make it
clear that many epileptics, whose stomachs are disordered by prolonged fasting, have fits from this very cause. Let us now suppose that
a patient is so plethoric that his arms, together with the parts round his
thighs and lower legs, are inflamed, and that the time of year is the
beginning of spring. This is not at all an improbable assumption, for we
have often seen patients affected in this way at that time. Let it be
further supposed that the person who is in such a state is unaccustomed to massage and exercises, and that he is harmed by fasting; then
let us enquire how we shall evacuate him. Shall it be with frequent
baths, or exercises, or with vomits after meals, or with fasting? for
these, according to Erasistratus, are the remedies for plethos. But he
himself does not think it right that those who are unaccustomed to
exercise should engage in it; and he excludes from baths all those who
are subject to[55] epileptic seizures. He will likewise, I think, exclude
them from vomits, since it is well known that they promote congestion
K244 of the head. And fasting by itself, in patients who are so plethoric as to
have a strong sensation of tension in the legs and arms, is inadequate
to evacuate them sufficiently, while it has the added disadvantage of
doing grave harm if the patient happens to have an easily disordered
stomach. How then shall we evacuate him? With massage alone,
which Erasistratus does not mention at all? But in patients who are
unaccustomed to it one cannot apply massage in such a way as to
evacuate adequately. Or shall we bind him with woollen bandages?
This is something that Erasistratus does not mention at all here,
although he does in his work on bringing up blood. Let us suppose,
however, that he did mention it, to make our enquiry as comprehen-
sive as possible. But it has been remarked earlier that this remedy was
not only troublesome but also ineffective in those who have come to
such a stage of plethora as to have a burning sensation in the limbs. I
cannot agree with what Erasistratus wrote in his book on bringing up
blood, namely that the danger of this condition is associated with the
danger of inflammation; and he contends that in this condition, when
one is making use of fasting, one ought not to reduce the patient's

the brain (K xv111a, 85). Thus in pain or grief, a bilious fluxion descends on it, since it
is weakened. In disease of the stomach the eyes may be suffused by sympathy (K v111,
139), and phantasmata or hallucinations may be generated (K v111, 221–4). The brain
is sympathetically affected by vapours rising from the stomach, and the mind
becomes disordered (K v111, 48–9). A variety of sympathetic symptoms, including
syncope, heartburn, dyspnoea, epilepsy, and melancholia, result from pathological
conditions at the cardiac orifice (K v11, 127–8).

55 A word or words meaning 'subject to' have been lost before the infinitive; Kotrc (1970)
inserts them.

strength by phlebotomy. For there is no necessity at all for inflam- K245
mation to follow plethora if we forestall it by evacuation. Yet even
when this plausible but false argument from his book on health is
abandoned, it is still true that Erasistratus did not dare to evacuate by
phlebotomy the plethos that is about to cause either epilepsy or
bringing up of blood. My proposition therefore is that he always
observed the exact doctrine of Chrysippus and used neither phlebotomy nor any of the powerfully purging drugs; for it is possible to
empty out the plethos both by means of phlebotomy and by some
kinds of purging. Erasistratus, however, has not written about them
here, nor in his books on paralysis and on gout. He blames plethora,
but uses neither phlebotomy nor any of the powerful purgatives. He
makes his own views even clearer in his book on bringing up blood, in
that part of the text where he says that some people run the risk of K246
bringing it up when their accustomed excretions are suppressed.
When he mentioned the removal of haemorrhoids[56] in dealing with
the other suppressions, he did not simply say that such patients
required evacuation, but described all the evacuant remedies of which
he approved, by categories as he did in his other books; yet he did not
include phlebotomy. The passage is as follows: 'In the patients in
question, who have been accustomed to losing[57] considerable
amounts of blood, excretion of both urine and sweat should be
encouraged. Limitation of food is also called for, and long slow walks
on the level.' In these remarks again we see him emptying out the
plethos with sweats, diuretics, fasting and walks, but not using
venesection. And indeed if he made it clear throughout this one book
that he did not use phlebotomy, whether before inflammation had
developed or when it was established or when it was expected to
occur, it would be superfluous for him to refer to phlebotomy in
another work, in which he treats of inflammation that is already K247
established, as in his book on fevers, or is about to begin, or
anticipated or actually beginning, as in his other works. But some of
the Erasistrateans, if they say he used phlebotomy as an evacuant
remedy, cannot see[58] any of these things; for the fact is, he has clearly
said the exact opposite. He says that, since it is no longer easy to give
food at the time when inflammation is occurring, he does not use
phlebotomy when inflammation is about to occur. This argument
shows directly that phlebotomy should be avoided in those patients in

---

[56] This may be a reference to the Hippocratic practice of keeping one pile intact (see
below, p. 124 n. 21); if this is not done, the patient will need evacuant treatment to
prevent unfortunate consequences.

[57] Reading ἔκκρισις for ἔκκλυσις; Kotrc (1970) does the same.

[58] Accepting Kotrc's (1970) emendation of ὁρῶσιν.

whom we plan to recommend fasting. It is not possible to use both remedies, fasting and phlebotomy, in one and the same patient; hence it is clear that whenever we find Erasistratus[59] advising fasting, he is not using phlebotomy at that time. This is why, as I said, he made no further mention of the remedy in his other works. In all of them, as I have shown, where he recommends fasting he quite clearly rejects

K248 phlebotomy. He is not acting correctly in this, as I have demonstrated earlier by quotations from each of the other books; yet he is less at fault than those who think that all those patients who need fasting automatically require phlebotomy. I shall therefore demonstrate in the succeeding work, not only that all patients do not require phlebotomy, but that even plethoric patients do not need it unless it has been previously established what the nature of the plethos is, and after that what the body type of the patient is, and his age and the season and the region and the prevailing circumstances, and the previous history and what is happening to him now. I shall show in respect of all these factors that many patients cannot undergo phlebotomy without harm. And in the same way again I shall show that many patients who have no plethora nevertheless require phlebotomy. As I deal with each of these matters I shall mention the proper time for phlebotomy and the amount; and, what is even more important, the differences between

K249 the veins that can be opened. The question of removing blood many times, as distinct from only once, will be considered, together with the no less important question whether one ought to bleed or purge, in spring, some people who are still in good health.[60]

---

[59] Reading Ἐρασίστρατον συμβουλεύοντα; so also Kotrc (1970).
[60] Accepting Kotrc's (1973) emendations of ἐπί τε τούτοις for ἐπί τε τούτων and ὥς τινας for ὥς τινες.

CHAPTER 4

Galeni de Curandi Ratione per Venae Sectionem
Galen's Book on Treatment by Venesection

This is a late work, in which Galen sums up his views on bloodletting at the request of colleagues who wanted something more manageable than his great work *On Therapeutic Method*.

Those who intend to use phlebotomy must consider first of all how many states of the body there are that call for evacuation. The next question is, which of these states require evacuation by phlebotomy; for there are many conditions, some of which need some other sort of evacuation, and certainly not bloodletting. The third problem is to decide which patients can stand the evacuation without harm, since sometimes the patient's condition demands phlebotomy, yet he cannot bear it either because of his stage of life, or the season of the K251 year, or the nature of the country, or because of some disorder of the mouth of the belly. (This is often miscalled the stomach; in the interests of brevity, however, I shall nevertheless use the term from now on in the whole of this work). There are also some who cannot bear phlebotomy because of their general habit of body, even though by reason of their disease they need it very much. If we are to draw such distinctions, we must consider each occasion[1] on its merits, just as we do with any other remedy. Our next question concerns the veins that are to be opened, since extensive research has been undertaken to decide whether it makes no difference which vein one chooses to cut, all being equally helpful in all conditions, or whether, as Hippocrates and the most celebrated physicians thought, it makes a great deal of difference whether one opens this one rather than that. When this has been settled, next comes the question of what one is aiming to achieve; by considering this one may estimate the quantity of the evacuation. And after all these, there is also the fact that in some patients it is better to remove blood only once, but in others to perform the operation known as epaphairesis; in some to evacuate to loss of consciousness, K252

---

[1] Reading, with La, καιρου for μέρους. Fu translates 'de occasione', and Ju, though translating 'particularis' as K's translator does, adds the note: 'Potius legendum περὶ καιροῦ, i.e. de occasione; sic ut videtur legisse antiquus interpres, qui semper καιρὸν vertit tempus.' The old translator he refers to may have been using La.

but in others to shun this as the greatest of evils. Anyone who wishes to use the remedy properly, then, must consider these matters.

2. All these things have already been dealt with in my book on therapeutic method, and also in a separate work against Erasistratus, which considers his mistaken rejection of the remedy. Then again there is another, against those Erasistrateans who maintain that the man did use it. One ends up not knowing whether to hate more[2] the wickedness of the accursed sophists, when they eagerly contrive new theories which they know perfectly well to be false, or their conceit of wisdom, when they make up arguments to discredit the most useful remedies, about which, in fact, they know nothing. Chrysippus the Cnidian fell into this second class, when he removed phlebotomy altogether from the list of medical remedies. His disciples Medius and Aristogenes followed him in this, and became famous among the Greeks. Erasistratus defended the doctrine of Chrysippus even more[3]
K253 stoutly, rising as a result to the most glittering heights of reputation. Next we have his own disciples, who all, initially at least, followed the dogma of their master, although later some revolted from it, being ashamed of their shameless shame.[4] How else can one describe the attitude of people who allege that Erasistratus approved of the remedy, when it is perfectly clear that nowhere in his works did he advise its use for any disease whatsoever? According to them, it is logical to suppose that anyone who used fasting as an evacuant remedy would naturally choose also to employ phlebotomy, since it is an even more effective one. Those who are of this opinion think it proper to phlebotomise all patients of the class for which Erasistratus ordered fasting to be used. So, since he wrote in his book on fevers, 'At the beginning of diseases, fasting', it follows that all should be phlebotomised; these people go so far as to argue thus on such occasions. It will indeed be a very great evil if those who are beginning their medical training are persuaded to act thus; but it will be worse still if they do not consider the other factors on which the decision
K254 should also be based. I have been obliged to discuss these in another work, to demonstrate to neophytes that Erasistratus did not use phlebotomy; for it is better that they should believe this than that they should phlebotomise every single one of those patients for whom Erasistratus ordered fasting. The book also shows that patients will derive the greatest benefit from the remedy when it is appropriately

---

[2] Literally 'On which account one might hate either ... or ...', but the sense seems to require the reading given.

[3] Reading ἔτι for ἐπὶ; suggested by an anonymous reader.

[4] αἰδεσθέντες ἀναίσχυντον αἰδῶ.

used. It did not seem necessary, therefore – to me at any rate – to write anything more about phlebotomy, since the use of the remedy has been discussed in my book on therapeutic method, as well as in my books on health, and in the two I wrote, one against Erasistratus himself, the other against the Erasistrateans in Rome, in which I drew attention to the wrong opinions he held. At the frequent request, however, of many friends in the profession, who seemed to me to have some aversion from reading *On Therapeutic Method*,[5] I was compelled in the end to undertake the present work, lest it should appear that I bore them some grudge, and to explain everything in order, appropriately set out, concerning the remedy. It is time, therefore, for me to begin my account.   K255

3. The word *diathesis*, as I have explained elsewhere,[6] is derived from διακεῖσθαι, and, like it, is predicated of many things. For the present at least, however, deviations towards the abnormal,[7] of whatever kind, will be referred to as diatheses in the whole of this work. We shall enquire, firstly, how many and what varieties of these deviations there are which call for evacuation, and secondly, which of these require phlebotomy. And since all objects of enquiry have two instruments of discovery – reason and experience – in all the arts, and for that matter in life in general, I think we ought to consider now whether the problem in hand is to be attacked by reason alone, or by experience alone, or by both. But since reason itself, starting from commonly held notions, not only discovers something[8] logically and so arrives at a proof, but also puts to use towards its demonstration the things it has learned in the course of these activities, and since we have seen that all the arts likewise use the methods of both reason and experience, we shall now apply whichever of them may prove to be useful. All men use the first of these methods in all the affairs of life, K256 but not all use the second,[9] for it is peculiar to those who practise the arts. The geometer demonstrates the first theorem of his art by the first

[5] Galen (K xv, 9), perhaps having a dig at colleagues who were put off by the size of this work, tells them how fortunate they are to have the book, which is of no small dimensions; in fact it fills a whole volume of Kühn (x, 1–1021) and must have been unmanageable in the days before indexing.

[6] K vii, 43, where Galen says that this derivation is approved by the old philosophers as well as the Greeks of his time. Since, as every schoolboy knows, it is in fact derived from διατίθημι, perhaps Galen's meaning is 'has become close in meaning to διακεῖσθαι'.

[7] Reading παρα φυσιν with the MSS. A diathesis, for Galen, is any stable condition of the body, not necessarily abnormal (K vii, 43). In this work Galen is concerned only with the diatheses that are abnormal. Such diatheses become diseases only if some bodily function is impaired. See E. H. Ackerknecht, 'Diathesis: the word and the concept in medical history', *Bull. Hist. Med.* 56 (1982) 317–25.

[8] Reading, with La, εὑρισκει τι.   [9] Galen seems to have reversed the order.

method only; thereafter he uses the second alone, and takes in addition towards his proof the conclusion he has drawn from the first. The further away he gets from his first theorem, the further he gets from his first method, and he ends up using it least of all. From the things he has proved he proves others, and from these others again, so that his proofs ultimately arrive at things unbelievable to the man in the street, not only the sizes of the sun, moon and earth, but also the knowledge of their distances.[10] Using these discoveries, those who follow this path make clocks and clepsydras and predict the eclipses of the sun and moon. Thus our argument, which is that of the arts, will use many things that have been demonstrated[11] in other works, including the fact that certain faculties[12] which govern the living creature are multiple, some being referred to as natural, others
K257 psychical.

All existing things have as their material of origin the four elements, whose nature it is to be altogether mingled among themselves and to act on one another. This being so, I shall make no further mention of Asclepiades in this work, since I have drawn attention to his false elements both in[13] the thirteenth commentary on the books of Demonstrations and in my work on the opinions of Asclepiades,[14] the fifth and sixth books of which include a refutation of his elements. The matter is also dealt with in my commentary on the elements of Hippocrates,[15] which concerns the effective qualities, namely heat, cold, dryness and dampness, and also the difference between the humours, and their genesis. I have also said a little about the drugs purging each of the humours in my book on the elements, and have dealt with them individually in another book. My book on temperaments,[16] which follows the work on the elements, is also useful in the present context. But the most valuable of all is the book on plethos,[17] in which I explain on one hand the dynamic form of plethos, and on the other the variety due to the dilatation of the space in which the
K258 liquid is contained. This kind is called by physicians plethos by filling.[18] Hence it is best for those who intend to study scientifically the

---

[10] Euclid, says Galen (K v, 654), proved by geometry that the earth is at the centre of the universe, but some philosophers dispute it, talking such nonsense as to make one ashamed of their whole profession. Galen's excessive reliance on logic in medicine is one of his most noticeable characteristics.

[11] Reading ἀποδεδειγμένοις, which may be the reading of the water-damaged La. I am indebted to Dr Nutton for confirming that the parts of this MS I have labelled illegible really are so.

[12] The natural faculties.   [13] Reading κατα τε with La.

[14] These works are lost. Asclepiades' elements would have been atoms and the void.

[15] K ɪ, 413–508.   [16] K ɪ, 509–694.   [17] K vɪɪ, 513–85.

[18] La has some words that are missing in K's Greek, though preserved in his Latin: ἐν ἦ περιεχεται τα ὑγρα καλειται δ' ὑπὸ τῶν ἰατρῶν . . .

matter of this book to have read my book on plethos; that book itself will indicate the preliminary reading that it in turn requires. No one should be surprised to hear that we need such preparation for a proper consideration of phlebotomy. For a knowledge of the books I have mentioned is necessary for finding out, not only about this remedy, but about all the others as well; so much so, indeed, that if it were possible, without a knowledge of these works, to treat patients correctly, I should not have gone to the trouble of writing them. It was necessary to say this by way of introduction.

Now it is time to begin the argument proper, by considering how many diatheses there are that require evacuation. If one merely enumerates them, having gathered them from one's experience, only to mention them is all the explanation needed. But if one goes by the logical way, it is necessary to find out what is common to all and universally present, and then by dissecting it into classes and differentia, as far as the ultimate varieties, to determine the number of conditions for which evacuation is indicated. Thus we shall demon- K259 strate all the conclusions that can be discovered by the way of logic.

4. The function of the art of medicine is both to restore all the natural functions of the parts of the body when they have been corrupted, and to preserve them once they have been restored. Now these corruptions follow upon the natural state; we must therefore both preserve this state while it is still in existence, and restore it when it has been corrupted. Since, then, it has been shown that the primary functions are effected by the homoiomerous parts, and the secondary ones by the organs, you ought to consider what beneficial or injurious effects the humours that are contained in the body may have on its parts. It has been shown in my book on plethos that plethos is of two kinds, both in origin and in terminology. One set of signs indicates dynamic plethos, another the variety due to dilatation of the vessels containing the humours, which some call plethos by filling. Both kinds call for evacuation, whether they occur in a sick man or in one in health. Just as a man who is carrying a load does not, as soon as he begins to feel K260 oppressed and tired, immediately fall down and concede defeat to it, so in the same way when the faculties are oppressed by plethos, it may be that the person has not yet become ill. If, then, some people who are still engaging in their usual occupations complain of feeling heavy, slow, lazy and sluggish, this is dynamic plethos. If, however, after exercise they seem to be distended, as Erasistratus said, and their upper arms and forearms are inflamed, this is an important indication of the other sort of plethos, which, as I have said, some call plethos by filling; for it comes about, and can be recognised, by humours being

poured into the vessels. I have pointed out in my books on health that
when an irritable sensation develops in the whole body, and particularly in relation to movement, such a state is the result of cacochymia.[19] But this too is commonly seen in those who are still going about
their customary duties. Signs may also appear in certain parts, rather
than in the whole mass, of the body, indicating conditions in those
K261 parts corresponding to those mentioned as affecting the whole body.
Thus we may have a feeling of heaviness, or some sort of ulcerous
sensation, which is confined to the head; or the temporal muscles may
be in spasm, either as an isolated condition or in association with an
increase in heat. Often, again, we have a sensation of weight in
relation to the liver, spleen, stomach, ribs or diaphragm; or sometimes, in the mouth of the belly, a feeling of weight, heartburn,
nausea, aversion from food, or perversion of appetite occurs. In
addition to these sensations, pains settling in any part, whether the
result of the concerted attack of a plethos of humours or of windy
pneuma, indicate the need for evacuation, as does acrid humour that
bites into a part and erodes it. Some pains originate from dyscrasia,
with or without an associated flux of humours. In all the conditions
just mentioned, the evacuation of the peccant humours or vapours
releases the patient from his sufferings, and phlebotomy is not needed
at all; it is enough to purge, rub and bathe him, and to anoint him with
K262 some diaphoretic drug. Now, however, we must explain in order what
are the conditions that are helped by phlebotomy.

5. Not only do the parts of the animal derive their nourishment from
the blood, but the innate heat also owes its continuance to it, just as
the fire on the hearth does to the burning of suitable logs, by which we
see whole houses made warm. And just as this fire is sometimes
harmed if faggots are piled on it indiscriminately, and sometimes if,
although not too abundant, they are very damp, or if none are put on it
at all, or very few – so also the heat in the heart sometimes becomes
less than normal because of the excess of blood, or a great shortage of
it, or a cold quality; and sometimes more, either because of a warm
quality of the blood, or a moderate excess of it. And whatever the heart
may suffer as a result of cold or heat, the other parts of the body
immediately share in. Sometimes unnatural heat or cold develops in
one particular part of the body, as has frequently been shown in other
K263 works. These conditions originate in two ways: sometimes as a result
of hot or cold humours, sometimes from dyscrasia alone. But these
localised states of heat and cold, when situated near to the affected
part, change with it; they do not extend to the whole body unless they

[19] K vi, 237. For the varieties of plethos see above, p. 12.

have first affected the heart. Similarly, it has been shown that the heart is affected in two ways: either as a result of dyscrasia, or else by hot and cold humours or a lack of one of these. I have shown that hot and cold humours are generated as a result of the quantity of food and drink that is taken, and of excessive ease or activity of the body and of the mind. Thus in the belly the digestive processes become disordered, and what is taken in becomes too phlegmatic or too bilious, or undergoes some other abnormal corruption, or remains raw and unconcocted for a long time, or is converted into flatus, so that the genesis of blood fails.[20] Analogous to these abortions of digestion in the belly are the states of the humours in the arteries and veins themselves. It is well known that anything hot and damp quickly K264 becomes rotten, particularly when in hot places; thus it must be that the nourishment distributed from the bowel, when it is not mastered by nature and changed into useful blood, will be liable to a different sort of putrefaction at another time. And since it is characteristic of things that rot from the heat of their matter to become hotter still, the blood that is putrefying will therefore be hotter, and when it has become so, the part in which it is rotting will itself be perceptibly warmer. And since the adjacent parts are heated at the same time by this perceptible heat, all the surrounding region will be heated, together with the parts thus affected, by the sharp and biting heat, since this is the nature of the heat from putrefaction. If, now, the part thus heated is an important one, capable of extending its own heat to the heart, either because it is near it, or is a vital organ, or because it is hot, it will heat that organ (the heart), inasmuch as the heart is very hot by nature. And once the heart is heated, the whole substance of it readily becomes hot, just as the house round the hearth is heated K265 when the hearth has a large fire on it. The Greeks call such a condition of the body fever. Sometimes the plethos of blood, before it has begun to putrefy, arrives in force at some part, either mortifying it completely, so as to destroy its function, or doing it notable damage. The apoplexies originate in this way, by a concerted rush of a quantity of blood to the governing centre of the animal. Similarly, when it descends on some other part, it causes an abnormal swelling in it. Inflammation also comes from this sort of process. When the blood that has descended on the part is too thick and melancholic, the swelling that results is scirrhous, just as it is flabby when the flux is more phlegmatic. When the flux is bilious it leads to erysipelas.[21] All

[20] For the innate heat and the genesis of the blood, see above, pp. 8–10; for putrefactive fevers, p. 12.
[21] See the work *On Abnormal Swellings*, above, p. 12, n. 48.

these things are precisely classified for you in the works I have recently mentioned. Now, as I said, applying the things that have been demonstrated to the question before us, I shall show that the argument concerning venesection follows from them. It seems best to start K266 from the fact that plethos is of two kinds. The variety known as dynamic plethos readily goes on to putrefy, and of course also sometimes descends on a part, causing abnormal swellings in parts so affected. The other sort, which is known as plethos by filling, also frequently rushes down into parts, leading to swellings, but it is a cause of apoplexies and rupture of veins as well; it is therefore essential to try to evacuate plethos quickly, before it has had a chance to do the patient some grave harm. How the two conditions are to be distinguished, and how to treat them, is described in more detail in my book on health;[22] similarly, when fever or bringing up of blood occur as a result of plethos or some of the apoplectic diseases, how to manage them is explained in my books on therapeutic method,[23] for which reason I consider it superfluous to write about them here. For if I were to write here too in the same way as I wrote in those works, I should have to go through the same subject in detail twice, and so prolong my discussion greatly. If, on the other hand, I were to make this account too brief, I should be in danger of suffering one of two K267 fates: either to express myself obscurely through brevity, or to omit some useful distinction. But since I did not undertake this work of my own volition, if anything I say in it should turn out to be mistaken, those who asked for it must bear the blame; just as, if it succeeds and proves to be useful, I shall give up the praise to them.

6. Now, therefore, let me take up my argument again. For those going about their normal activities, who have a sense of heaviness or of tension, either in one of the vital parts or in the whole body, evacuation is necessary. And if, where stage of life is concerned, they are no longer children nor have they already reached old age, consider phlebotomy, paying particular attention to the following primary indications. First come the amount of the plethos and its quality, and the strength or weakness of the faculties; then the physical type of the whole body, the season and the region and the patient's previous way of life, and whether he has taken an excess of food or drink, and particularly of nourishing food; whether this is habitual for him or contrary to custom; what exercise he has taken, what evacuations he K268 has had, or whether any have been held back contrary to habit; and in

---

[22] This is the work *De Sanitate Tuenda*, K vi, 1–452. R. M. Green has published an English version (*A translation of Galen's Hygiene*, 1951).
[23] *De Methodo Medendi*, K x, 1–1021.

addition to all these, whether he has become thinner or fatter. The quantity of any plethos is estimated from the magnitude of its characteristic signs. To whatever extent the patient has a sensation of heaviness, it is clear that dynamic plethos has increased to that degree; similarly, to whatever extent the sensation of tension has increased, to that extent also the other kind of plethos has increased, which, as I said, is called by some plethos by filling.[24] The quality – and this applies to both varieties of plethos – you will distinguish by the colour, bearing in mind that colours are characteristic of the humours[25] provided that the whole body is in a temperate state with respect to external heat and cold, and particularly with respect to those qualities that are part of the nature of the particular humour concerned.[26] This is because the whole body feels colder when the environmental conditions are colder, and warmer when they are warmer; swelling and distension[27] of the vessels follow the crowding of humours into

[24] The essence of dynamic plethos is that the faculties are weak, so that the peccant humour oppresses them; hence the sensation of weight. The other variety, plethos by filling, physically distends the vessels, so that the patient feels swollen.

[25] The author of On the Cosmos, a work probably of the first century AD falsely attributed to Aristotle, says (v, 396b) that painting uses the four colours red, white, blue and yellow, mixing them to represent all the colours of nature, just as in the universe the four elements are harmoniously mingled, and in music there is a eucrasia of high and low tones. He probably has eucrasia of the bodily humours in mind, since these are their colours, except that for Galen black bile is dark or leaden-coloured rather than blue.

[26] K's text ('provided that...' to 'humour concerned') reads ἐπειδὰν μετρίως ἔχει θερμότητος λείπων σῶμα φύσει and is clearly corrupt. La reads ἐπειδαν μετριως ἔχει θερμοτητος τε και ψυχροτητος της ἔξωθεν ὁλον το σωμα και προσετι των συνυπαρχοντων τη του χυμου φυσει.

Fuchsius, in his interesting commentary, observes: 'Animadvertendum etiam hoc loco erit, Graecum codicem non tantum esse depravatum, sed & mutilum. Emendandus vero erit hunc in modum': and he quotes the Greek of La exactly, except for the addition of ἐκ before τῶν συνυπαρχοντων. 'Cui quidem lectioni nostra per omnia respondet conversio. Et hanc plane esse legitimam antiquus interpres confirmat, qui praesentem locum ita reddidit: Quando moderate se habet in caliditate & frigiditate extrinseca totum corpus, & adhuc ex iis quae coexistunt humoris naturae.' His own translation reads 'siquidem universum corpus in calore & frigore externo mediocriter se habeat, partim ex iis quae humorum naturae insunt.' K's Latin translation reproduces that of Gaudanus, except that it has colore for calore, and adds totum before corpus, following here Ju, which is a modified version of Gaudanus. It seems remarkable that Fuchsius, without possessing the correct Greek text, could have reproduced it so exactly from the Latin version of the 'antiquus interpres', who, it again appears, used La or a closely related MS. The Aldine reads ἐπειδὰν μετρίως ἔχει θερμότητός τε καὶ ψυχρότητος σῶμα*φύσει; the asterisk is its customary alternative to the crux. Ch is identical with K.

I think the meaning of the sentence is that the identity of the humour comprising the plethos can be determined from the colour of the body, provided that the body is not too hot or cold because of the state of its environment. Too hot an environment might cause one to think that the humour concerned was a warm one (bile or blood) and too cold an environment that it was cold (black bile or phlegm).

[27] Reading διατασις with A, U, M, K's translator, Ju and Fu; Ga, however, has read διάθεσις with K (affectio).

the veins, while where the flesh is involved a sensation either of weight or of tension follows, and indeed also of heat. It has been shown that the weakness or strength of the faculties that govern us is K269 to be judged from the activities proper to them. The faculties in the nerves, and in their origin, the brain, are assessed by the state of the deliberative functions, and those in the arteries and heart by the pulse, while by the good or poor state of nutrition and by the good colour or pallor of the complexion the decision is made concerning the third faculty, the nutritive, which I have shown to proceed from the liver.[28] When, therefore, signs of plethos are present and the faculties are in good condition, you will obviously phlebotomise, taking no other factors into consideration when you are dealing with a condition marked by distension; and this applies even more strongly if there is inflammation. But where there is heavy oppression by plethos it is not always desirable to remove blood. It is possible for crude humour[29] to collect in the body, in which event it is necessary to consider precisely, not only to what extent the faculties are in good condition, but also to what extent the humour has increased. For when the faculties have already been broken up by such conditions, they are liable, if phlebotomy is used, to sink to their last extremity, so that it is no longer possible to restore them. When this happens the danger is great, and particularly when, in warm weather, there is an attack of fever while the stomach is disordered, or when the whole body is by nature soft K270 and damp in its temperament. Patients of this sort quickly become weakened and worn out, even if a powerful fever does not attack them. If none of these things happens, but it is winter, or the region is naturally cold, or the nature of the patient is rather cold, those who are phlebotomised suffer dreadfully from chilling of the whole body, and the patient falls into one of the troubles that follow severe chilling. Patients in this condition ought not to be evacuated by phlebotomy, but rather with rubbings and anointings that warm moderately, and drinks that cut through the glutinosity[30] of the humours and have a moderate warming effect. Preparations that heat powerfully dissolve the faculties too suddenly, and are thus unsuitable for continuous treatment; besides, they often increase the fever at the same time, so that damage is done from this cause too to the faculties. For the same

[28] It is extremely important to estimate the strength of the main governing faculties of the body, which proceed from the three divisions of the Platonic soul (see above, pp. 5–6). Where venesection is concerned, those seated in the heart are the most important; hence the significance of the pulse.

[29] Crude or raw humour is material, derived from nutriment, that has not been properly cooked or concocted by the innate heat.

[30] Crude humour is glutinous because, being undercooked, it is cold.

reason the heating effect of foods and drinks that break up the thickness of the humours ought to be moderate.

7. Those who have been temporarily cured by spitting blood, but nevertheless have a condition in the parts round the chest and lungs by virtue of which, if a slightly increased amount of blood should K271 accumulate in them,[31] some vessel will again have its mouth forced open or be ruptured – these patients must be phlebotomised at the beginning of spring,[32] even if there are as yet no symptoms anywhere in the body. The same applies to those who fall readily into fits, and to apoplectics. In the same way, if we know that the patient is susceptible to some other disease, for instance a peripneumonic, pleuritic or synanchic condition, it is better to phlebotomise in advance rather than wait for some clear sign of plethos to show itself. This applies also to those in whom haemorrhoids have been suppressed, and particularly if they appear somewhat melancholic. And as for those who go down every year in summer with plethoric diseases, they too should be evacuated at the onset of spring. Similarly those who are seized in spring itself with such diseases, some having weak eyes, or being subject to the diseases called scotomatic – these also need to be evacuated at the beginning of spring, after we have first considered what sort of concourse of humours they have. This is because some accumulate the bilious humour more than the rest, others the melan- K272 cholic or phlegmatic variety, while others again accumulate all of them equally; in these, blood is said to be in excess.[33] You will evacuate all these, as you will also your gouty and arthritic patients, at the beginning of spring, either by purging or by phlebotomising. I have cured many who had already been troubled on and off for two or three years with pains in the feet, either purging away the excessive humour at the beginning of spring, or removing blood. It is clear that such people are of the sort who are temperate in their way of life, because you will not help the immoderate winebibbers and gluttons much by purging or phlebotomising them; they quickly accumulate a mass of crude humours through intemperate living. One really ought not to undertake to treat these patients;[34] but where they are cooperative,

---

31 Reading, with La, ὡς εἰ βραχυ ἀθροισθείη το αἷμα.
32 Prophylactic venesection is undertaken in spring because this is the season in which blood predominates, as we know from *Nature of Man*, the foundation of Galen's humoral system (L 6, 46). In summer bile, a more dangerous humour, predominates, and ancient medicine was far more concerned than we are today with preventing disease while the patient was still in health.
33 Because blood is the only well-tempered humour; see above, pp. 7–8.
34 The ancient physician evidently felt no obligation to accept a patient who consulted him. The Hippocratic work *On the Art* (L 6, 4–6, 14) makes it clear that in those times the physician did not undertake to treat hopeless cases; as Plato (*Republic* II, 360e)

you will help them most at the beginning of spring, first evacuating them in advance, and then leading them on to exercises and a healthy way of life. You must consider what I have said of these patients to apply also to those who are liable to be seized with the diseases I have just mentioned, such as epilepsy, apoplexy, scotomatic diseases, haemoptysis and melancholy.

K273   8. Not only is phlebotomy of great benefit in the presence of plethos, either of the dynamic variety or of the kind known as plethos by filling, but it is useful also when inflammation is beginning in the absence of plethos, as a result either of a blow, or pain, or atony of the parts; for the pain attracts blood to it, and frequently laxity of the parts leads to inflammation in the absence of plethos of the whole body. It was shown in my works on the natural faculties that when a part is naturally weak it at once becomes heavy, even if only a small amount of residue should collect in it. And of course it is also true that every part has a faculty by which it attracts things proper to it; it follows, therefore, that it must also have another for excreting things that are foreign, and that this foreignness is twofold, one kind of material being foreign by reason of its quantity, the other by its quality. For this reason, if some part is not weighed down by the humours in it, but nevertheless contains some residues which are abnormal in respect of
K274   quality, it hastens to excrete them through the veins in it, as if through conduits. Now whether the material thus expelled is bad blood, or some other humour, it must arrive at some nearby part. In this part, one of two things can happen. If the humour is digested or corrupted, it does not flow across to a third part; but if neither of these things befalls it, it can flow again, from the second part to another, and from that part in turn to still another one; and this process does not cease until it descends on some part that is of such a kind that it cannot thrust the excess in it through to another part. This happens to those parts that have the weakest excretory powers of all the parts in the vicinity. They can no longer eject the troublesome matter into other parts, since these do not accept it by reason of the strength in them. I have shown in those commentaries, not only that each part pushes the excess towards its neighbour, but that sometimes the adjacent part accepts it, and at other times sends it back and repels it without receiving it into itself, and in this contest the strongest part wins. This

---

says, the skilful pilot or physician knows what is impossible in his art and what possible, and attempts the one and not the other. The doctor, Galen says in the *De Methodo Medendi*, should not treat patients who are already marasmic; and in hectic fevers, where marasmus has not yet set in, the relatives should be warned of the danger (K x, 720–1). The ancient physician was more concerned with maintaining his reputation than his modern counterpart is.

is why the weakeśt parts of all are the first to be seized with diseases due to residues.[35] You may know that the diseases known as rheumatic also originate in a somewhat similar way. When the whole body is K275 weak, which is one of the signs of cachexia,[36] the vital parts of it are liable to be weighed down, and even if there is not much blood in them, this is pushed through to the fleshy parts near the skin, and particularly into the glands that are adapted to receive the excess through the porosity of their substance and because they have weaker natural faculties than the other parts have. This is true also of the fat.[37] As I have shown, there are four of these faculties: first the attractive, second the retentive, third the excretory, and fourth the transformative.[38] The glands and the flesh have the other three very weak, and only the transformative faculty not much inferior to the other parts. Next to the glands the lung[39] is the most ready to receive the flow, since this organ has the three powers weak, and its substance is porous. Next comes the spleen. The brain is similar to these, or perhaps even better adapted to receive the flow. It has the advantage of them by reason of its structure, which is adapted for the excretion of K276 what it has received, for it has capacious ventricles discharging by downward passages. In those people in whom the lung, spleen and brain are stronger than the fleshy parts, the fluxions go to the glands and flesh, with weakening of the whole constitution of the body, as happens in the rheumatic diseases. Naturally, therefore, the aim of treatment is not evacuation, but strengthening of the whole body; in spite of this, however, treatment for these patients begins with bloodletting. When the residues are troublesome by reason of their quality we also use purgation, chiefly on those bodies in which we are not awaiting the appearance of the characteristic signs of either kind of plethos, namely weight for dynamic plethos, tension for the variety from filling. In the same way, when some part has been severely bruised, or is for some other reason the seat of incipient inflammation, whenever we expect this inflammation to be severe we begin the treatment with evacuation, either purging or phlebotomising, whichever we think will provide it better. K277

---

[35] For the movement of residues, see above, p. 11.

[36] Cachexia, according to Celsus (III.22.1–3) is a variety of wasting; because of the bad state of the body, resulting from chronic disease, improper treatment or wrong diet, everything taken in is corrupted. Skin eruptions are frequent, and some parts may become swollen.

[37] For the glands and brain, and the probable origin of Galen's beliefs, see the Hippocratic work *Glands* (L 8, 556–74).

[38] Galen's work on the natural faculties, K II, 1–214, has already been referred to (above, p. 3, n. 6).

[39] Hence the danger of pleurisy, peripneumonia and phthisis when there are residues at large in the body.

9. Rightly, then, in the appendix[40] to the books on regimen in acute diseases we are exhorted to use phlebotomy when the disease is severe and the patient in the prime of life and strong. And Menodotus[41] is wrong in saying that phlebotomy should be approved only in the syndrome known as the plethoric. Quite the reverse; the indications for phlebotomy do not primarily include plethos, but the suspicion that disease is developing. If it appears that it will be severe, we shall invariably phlebotomise, even if none of the signs of plethos is present, having regard to the patient's age and the region and his faculties, which are the only factors to be mentioned in the appendix to the book on regimen. The author mentioned the man in the prime of life to distinguish him from children and the aged; the first and most important indications for phlebotomy are, however, the severity of the disease and the strength of the patient, and it is necessary to say that this, and not the plethoric syndrome, is the principal combination of circumstances for which phlebotomy has always been approved. For the syndrome that increases the severity of the disease is also included among the indications;[42] the time for phlebotomy is not only when

[40] I read προσκειμένοις with K's Latin translator. There seems no doubt about the correctness of this, since the passage in question (L 2, 398) occurs only in the *Appendix* to *Regimen in Acute Diseases*. All the MSS, however, as well as Ald and Ch, read προκειμενοις, both here and in line 11, and again at 278, line 15, where, unless they are all in error, the meaning can only be (because of the preposition ἐν) 'the propositions set forth in *Regimen in Acute Diseases*'. La reads (at 277, line 1) ἐν τοις προκειμενοις κἀν τῷ περι διαιτης ὀξεων which most probably means 'in the foregoing and in *Regimen in Acute Diseases*'. Ju's Latin agrees (as usual) with K's; but Ga has 'Recte ergo admonemur in iis qui exempli causa in libro de ratione victus acutorum proponuntur', and Fu 'Recte igitur in iis quae de victu acutorum morborum proposita & disputata sunt admonemur.'
      For further discussion of this *Appendix* see below, pp. 115–18.

[41] Menodotus (probably second century AD) the Empiricist. According to Galen, he had confuted Asclepiades, who paid no attention to facts. The plethoric syndrome comprised distension of the veins, redness and heaviness of the whole body, sluggishness of movement, and a feeling of tension in the limbs, together with, according to some, a sensation of irritation, pain or lassitude, a previous history of physical inactivity and of excess of food or drink, and suppression of some wonted evacuation (K VII, 515–16). This is a mixed bag of signs and symptoms of the two varieties of plethos, together with some, such as the ulcerous or irritating sensation, that are, according to Galen, not symptoms of plethos at all, but of qualitative cacochymia due to biting humours, and of weakness of the faculties (K VII, 547–8, 554, 561).
      Galen says Menodotus wrote that the goal of the physician was fame and profit; but Diocles, Hippocrates and Empedocles took a different view, and practised for the love of humanity (K V, 751–2). For Galen's views of Hippocrates, see the work *That the Best Physician is also a Philosopher*, referred to on p. 1. One of the most famous of the Hippocratic precepts urges the physician to give his services to the poor without charge, 'for where the love of man is, there also is the love of this Art' (L 9, 258).

[42] Galen's meaning is somewhat obscure here. It seems to be that phlebotomy is called for when the signs and symptoms suggest that severe disease will occur in the near future, although it is not yet present; Menodotus would have used it only where the full-blown plethoric syndrome was already established.

severe disease is already established, but also whenever it is likely to K278
occur. The doctrine Hippocrates enunciated for our instruction has
anticipated us; it teaches us that however much we may rightly do
once diseases are already present, it is nevertheless better for us to
forestall them by action when they are beginning, or about to begin.
Thus it is possible to carry over the indications mentioned, and apply
them to people in health. You will phlebotomise these people too
when it becomes probable that they will be seized with a severe[43]
disease, taking into consideration their age and their strength; since if
someone is liable to suffer from a severe disease, even if no sign of it
yet exists anywhere in the body, we think it proper to perform
phlebotomy. It is enough to take into consideration the patient's age,
together with his strength, so that the three factors upon which the
decision is made are the severity of the disease, whether present or
expected; the stage of life in the prime, and the strength of the
faculties. Perhaps the matter of stage of life may seem to be explained
rather carelessly in the appendix to the book on regimen in acute
diseases. It is wrong to mention the prime of life alone; one should
refer also to the time before it and the time after it, as otherwise two
periods, that of childhood and that of old age, would be excluded from K279
the distinction. The period of age, however, can be excluded under the
heading of strength, since none is strong at that stage of life. Some
physicians have thought that strength was likewise absent in children,
but they judged wrongly, as I have shown in other works. We shall
phlebotomise, then, if we expect the disease to be severe, or if we see
that it already exists or is starting, taking into consideration the
strength of the faculties; we shall except only children from the rule,
and we shall say that the distinction on the grounds of age drawn by
the author of the appendix to *Regimen in Acute Diseases* was rather
inadequately expressed. These indications for phlebotomy are all that
is needed. When a plethos of crude humours has accumulated to such
an extent as to call for phlebotomy, the rule is not broken, since such
patients lack strength of the faculties. The sign that patients are unable
to bear phlebotomy is this: the complexion of the whole body lacks[44]
the colour that indicates an abundance of blood, and at the same time
the pulse shows an abnormality in respect of force and of volume,
characterised by a predominance of feeble and small beats.   K280

---

[43] La has an illegible word between μεγαλω and μηδεν. A is quite illegible here, and has a
crux in the margin. U and M both have a space after μεγαλω, followed by διο καν. The
corruption perhaps goes back to a common ancestor of La and A, which must have
been at several removes because of the widely different readings frequently offered
by these two MSS.

[44] Reading ἐκπεπτωκοτι with La and K's Latin translator.

Now that we have defined three indications for phlebotomy, namely the severity of the disease, whether existing, expected, or beginning; age in the prime of life; and strength of the faculties, childhood excepted, we come to the other criteria for phlebotomy I have recently mentioned, which many doctors have added, indicating the amount to be removed, not whether phlebotomy itself should be undertaken. This is because the decision that one ought to let blood is made from the disease and the time of life and the strength, while the amount of the evacuation is not decided from these alone, but by taking the others into consideration also. These are the syndrome known as the plethoric, and the temperament of the air surrounding us, classified according to season and region; the events of the patient's past life in respect of the quality and quantity of food; whether or not his excretions have occurred, and whether he has taken exercise. We shall look into these distinctions a little later.

10. I shall deal with the distinguishing features of either kind of plethos in the present work, considering whether we shall invariably have recourse to phlebotomy whenever these signs appear in K281 someone who is still going about his ordinary activities, or whether this is not obligatory when there is no expectation of grave disease. But whatever my opinion on this may be, you know that you yourselves have often been with me when I have recommended venesection for gouty patients, or arthritics, epileptics, melancholics, or those with a history of haemoptysis, or a condition in the chest predisposing to such a disease, or scotomatics,[45] or those who are repeatedly seized with synanche or peripneumonia, or pleurisies, or liver diseases, or severe attacks of ophthalmia; in fact, to speak generally, with any severe disease. I say that in all such conditions phlebotomy is an essential remedy that must be applied immediately, as long as the patient's strength and age are also taken into account. These factors, even if sometimes not specifically mentioned, must be taken for granted. And for those patients who have never suffered from any such disease before, because they have all the parts of their bodies faultlessly constructed, you probably know that I propose a twofold way of evacuation: by phlebotomy if they are intemperate in their way of life, without it if they are temperate. This is because it is possible to clear out the plethos quickly with frequent rubbings, baths, walks and K282 other exercises, and further with diaphoretic anointings, unless, of course, it should appear to you that there is an excess of thick blood.

[45] Scotomatic disease (σκότος, darkness) was characterised by giddiness and falling; as we say, 'blackouts'. It might be due to trouble at the cardiac orifice of the stomach (K VIII, 204).

Such a plethos is usually mostly melancholic, though occasionally it also contains some admixture of what are called crude humours. In the condition known as melancholic excess it is better to phlebotomise than to rely solely on a drug purging black bile.[46] When crude humours prevail, however, evacuate cautiously before the patient begins to sicken; but if, as I have mentioned before, he is already feverish, do not evacuate at all. You will have an indication of these humours in the leaden tint of the complexion, or a yellowish white[47] shade, or anything other than red, and in the irregularity of the pulse. If a plethos of these humours has undergone sufficient development, there is, in addition to these signs, a sense of heaviness of the body and tiredness on exertion, with mental sluggishness and a dulling of consciousness. On the other hand you should phlebotomise boldly those who have accumulated blood through suppression of haemorrhoids, even if they have no previous history of severe disease; for it is possible that they are in fact susceptible to some such disease, though they have never yet suffered from it because of the evacuation through K283 the haemorrhoids. And if they appear further to be deformed in some part, and in particular a part of the chest,[48] you will phlebotomise them for certain, without delay.

11. You know that I have the same opinion concerning women whose menstrual purgation has been suppressed. Evacuation should not be deferred in these patients either; it is not essential, however, to open a vein, for in fact scarifications of the ankles are sufficient to eliminate the excess, since they possess some other power to urge on the menstrual changes, just as venesections at the ankles and hams do. You should always evacuate women who suffer from suppression of the menses from the legs, either by opening a vein or by scarifying. Phlebotomy at the elbow is liable to suppress the purgations of women. Those of them who are of fairer complexion collect thinner blood, and hence derive the greatest benefit from scarification at the ankles. But treat those who are darker by phlebotomy, since they accumulate thicker and more melancholic blood, particularly if they appear to have larger veins; these are found in the more slender and K284 darker women, while smallness of the veins is characteristic of those who are plump and fair, and in these it is better to scarify the ankles than to cut a vein. And indeed these women have small veins in their legs, so that the right amount does not escape even if they are well

---

[46] Galen believed that particular drugs purged specific humours; see n. 53 below.
[47] Reading ὠχρολευκον with La.
[48] Because of the danger of a concourse of humours settling in the chest, which is more likely to happen if it is weak.

phlebotomised.[49] You ought not to despise phlebotomy as a revulsive remedy, since you have often seen me, when there is a copious haemorrhage from the nostrils, making use of the remedy and stanching the flow forthwith. It is expedient, then, as you have seen, not to delay until the patient's strength has reached the last stages of collapse, but, when it appears that the appropriate amount has been evacuated, and the force of the rush of blood continues strong, to cut a vein at the elbow, in the right arm if the right nostril is bleeding, in the other side for the left one. At the same time as you do this, apply bandages of fillet-material to the limbs, and a cupping-glass to the hypochondrium on the affected side.[50] When we do this, as you know, we invariably check the haemorrhage from the nostrils, in spite

K285 of having previously tried the drugs recommended in the literature for stuffing up the nose[51] and rubbing on the forehead, and found them all ineffective. Thus, in addition to what was said previously about phlebotomy, this too overthrows the theory of Menodotus,[52] who believed that the syndrome known as plethoric would put us in mind of the remedy. The condition now under discussion is clearly the opposite of plethoric; we use venesection for it, not as an evacuant, but as a revulsive remedy.

12. Nothing shows so clearly that the medical art is in practice a matter of guesswork as the question of the amount of each remedy. We often know exactly that the time for administering food or drink, whether cold or hot, is at hand; we cannot be sure, however, of how much we ought to give. It is the same with purgatives; we sometimes know for certain that a drug purging yellow bile, black bile, phlegm or serous superfluities[53] should be given to the patient; yet we do not

---

[49] Body type is very important in Galen's system, since it indicates both the general crasis of the patient and also the temperament of individual parts. As far as the veins are concerned, Galen says in his work *De Temperamentis* that people with broader veins are hotter by nature, and are thus dark and slender; if a fat person has broad veins, he is not naturally fat, but has become so by his mode of life. Those with broad veins also have more blood, and bear fasting better than those with colder natures, who tend to be plump and fair, with narrow veins and little blood. Women tend to be fatter on the whole than men because they are colder by nature, and more sedentary in their way of life (K I, 604–6). See also section 13, this work, K 289f.

[50] Galen's rationale for undertaking revulsive venesections from particular sites and sides of the body is discussed in Chapter 8 below.

[51] Reading ἐντιθεμένων with all the MSS and K's Latin translator.

[52] See n. 41 above.

[53] Specific drugs purge specific humours, in Galen's system, because, being derived from living things, they have the attractive faculty, by which they draw what is similar to themselves. The materialist Asclepiades disagreed, since he denied the natural faculties. In his system, since everything in creation was made up of atoms and the passages in which they moved, nothing could be either cognate or foreign to the body; quantity, not quality, was the only cause of trouble, and the treatment for an excess of anything was merely to reduce the patient's diet. Galen, however, held

know with any certainty[54] the amount that should be administered. A K286
dose[55] of such preparations cannot be corrected. Once the drug has
been swallowed and has entered the belly it must of necessity all be
digested; nor can one, if the patient has already been purged more
than is desirable, remove any part of what has been administered. The
greatest advantage of phlebotomy is that you can stop the evacuation
whenever you wish, and afterwards at any time you choose allow it to
flow again up to whatever quantity may seem good to you. Hence it is
better, if there is no urgency, to make the first bloodletting rather
small, and to perform a second one[56] – and, if you like, a third – later.
Thus in cases where extensive evacuation is called for, but the faculties
are not strong, it is appropriate to divide up the evacuation, as you
must have seen me doing in patients who have a plethos of somewhat
crude humours. After I have let a little blood I immediately give some
melicratum, nicely cooked, with one of the attenuating drugs, hyssop
or organy or even mint or pennyroyal; one may also give oxymel or
oxyglycy with melicratum.[57] After this I take blood again, sometimes
on the same day, sometimes on the next; at which time I again give one K287
of the drugs mentioned, in the same way, and remove blood once
more; and on the third day I repeat the same process twice. When,
however, there is a plethos of seething blood, enkindling a very acute
fever, there is need for copious evacuation. One must try to evacuate
this blood to the point of fainting, keeping an eye on the strength of
the faculties. I know, for instance, of some doctors who take six
cotyles,[58] either all at once or spread over two, three or four days, and
sometimes on the very first day of the illness, in cases where fever had
set in about nightfall or in the course of the night, and the food taken
the previous day had been well digested. I know that I myself have let
blood at the end of the first day in some patients who attributed
sweating, or pain in the head or some other part, to an indisposition of
the previous day, and for this reason took too little food, and were
beginning to be feverish as night came on. For in those patients who
appear to you to have a plethos of seething blood, you must try to
evacuate it as quickly as possible, before it descends on some vital part;

that if a drug purging, say, phlegm was given to a patient suffering from an excess of
bile, it would purge very little bile and do grave harm; a drug specifically attracting
bile, however, would do good (K I, 497–500).

[54] La has the word βεβαιως, which I translate, after ἐπιστάμεθα.

[55] Reading δοσις with A, U and M. All these MSS leave out ἀλλὰ τοιαύτη, and La is
illegible.

[56] This is the procedure of epaphairesis (repeated removal).

[57] Melicratum was a mixture of honey and water, or perhaps milk. Oxymel and
oxyglycy were made from honey and vinegar.

[58] About 1,700 ml, or almost half the total blood volume of a small adult.

hence you will not shrink from sometimes opening a vein even during
K288 the night. What most people do, letting blood only between the
second hour of the day and the fourth or fifth, is laughable; if it were
not that I have seen them giving enemas, food and other remedies at
any time of the night, I should have some hard things to say to them.
Since, however, they do not observe one and the same restricted
period of hours for everything they do for all their patients, but act as
the disease requires, awaiting the time just mentioned only in the case
of phlebotomy, their error is easier to excuse.

It is appropriate to take patients in this condition, as I have said, as
far as loss of consciousness. I have seen some of them, from the
chilling that invariably accompanies fainting, sweat from the whole
body and pass faeces, after which they quickly recover from their
disease.[59] It is good, however, to pay attention to the diminution of the
pulse, feeling it while the blood is still flowing, as is usually done in all
patients who are being phlebotomised, so that you will never negli-
gently cause your patient death instead of loss of consciousness, a
K289 thing I know has happened to three doctors. One of them phlebotomised a feverish woman, and each of the others a man, into such a
deep faint that they could not be resuscitated. For this reason it is
better to avoid copious evacuations unless some great necessity
demands them. And moreover revulsion, a remedy of no small
importance and one that is often effected by phlebotomy, becomes
more effective in proportion as you increase the number of separate
bloodlettings from different parts. It is better to know this in advance.

13. Recapitulating from the beginning the subject before us, let us
now consider what we know to be the most essential for those who
wish to practise phlebotomy without ever doing harm. First one must
know that the indications for the remedy, which have been mentioned, show the need for a larger evacuation when they are increasing; when they are becoming feebler, however, they show that one
should reduce the evacuation proportionately with their decline. The
severity of the disease, then, together with the strength of the
faculties, were the chief indications for phlebotomy: the former by
showing what must be done, the latter by not prohibiting it. (This is
K290 what some of the newer physicians call a contraindication.) For there
are times when the patient's condition demands phlebotomy, but the

---

[59] In the *De Methodo Medendi* Galen says that in continuous fevers, bloodletting to the
point of fainting cools the body greatly, extinguishing the fever forthwith. Nothing
could be more pleasant, both to the patient and to the nature that governs living
things. He recalls a case in which, after he had performed one of these heroic
evacuations, the bystanders exclaimed 'Man, you have slaughtered the fever!', at
which, he says, 'we all laughed' (K x, 612).

weakness of the faculties forbids it. When both of these indications require it, it is, as mentioned earlier, clearly called for, as long as there is no plethos of crude humours in such quantity and of such a kind as to prohibit the use of the remedy. Next, we must consider together with these indications what sort of natural temperament the person has. Those who have large veins, who are moderately slender and neither fair nor soft-fleshed, you will evacuate freely. Those of the opposite type, however, must be sparingly evacuated, since they have little blood and flesh that transpires well.[60] For the same reason you will not phlebotomise children up to the age of fourteen. After this age, if at any time blood should appear to be accumulating in large quantities, and the time of year is spring and the region temperate, and the nature of the child abounding in blood, you will let blood, especially if there is a lurking danger of peripneumonia, synanche, or pleurisy, or some other acute and severe disease. Generally you will take up to one cotyle of blood at the first operation; if, after this, you find on examining the patient that the strong state of the faculties is K291 being maintained, you will add a further half by way of epaphairesis. You have learned to trust the strong, regular pulse as an infallible sign of strength of the faculties; this applies even more strongly to the large pulse. Thus you will phlebotomise even the seventy-year-olds, if the kind of pulse I have mentioned is present, whenever their condition demands it. Even at this time of life there are still some full-blooded people whose powers are at the same time strong, just as there are others who are dried up and have little blood and bruise easily when any part is injured by a blow.[61] Hence you will not take into account only the sum of years, as some do, but also the habit of the body. Some sixty-year-olds can no longer bear phlebotomy, while some people of seventy still can. But obviously you will remove less from these, even if they appear to be in the same condition as a body in the prime of life.

14. It is best to consider all these matters before cutting a vein, and particularly to think about suppressed haemorrhoids and the menstrual catharsis. Once the vein has been cut and there is a flow of

---

[60] See also n. 49 above. The Hippocratic work *Diseases of Women* II gives further information on these physical types (L 8, 238–40).

[61] The text is corrupt, but the meaning seems clear. K's Greek, μελαινόμενοι, is not followed by his Latin translator, who read μαραινόμενοι and rendered it *arescentes*. All the MSS agree here with K's Greek. A marginal note in Ju attributes the reading *nigrescentes*, which it correctly says is that of the Aldine, to Oribasius. Fuchsius again enlists the help of his old translator: '& in partibus corporis percussi facile nigrescentes. Sic enim legendum, quum in greco sit μελαινόμενοι, non arescentes, ut alius interpres convertit, qui legit μαραινόμενοι. Quam quidem lectionem etiam antiquus confirmat interpres, qui hoc loco convertit facile nigrescentes.'

K292 blood, it is necessary to consider the change in it, particularly when there is already inflammation, the reduction in the tone of the flow, and most of all the change in the pulse. This is an infallible[62] sign, and you must stop the bleeding immediately if it changes, either in volume or by developing any sort of abnormality. What more is there to say about the change towards indistinctness, since you have learned that in this quality there is a sound criterion of the strength, as well as the weakness, of the faculties? In patients who have a large inflammatory focus near the vein that has been opened, it is best to await a change both in the colour and in the consistency of the blood, as Hippocrates has also explained in his book *Regimen in Acute Diseases*, speaking of pleurisy. The blood in inflammation is different from the normal variety, being greatly overheated. If it was previously cruder, it becomes redder and yellower; if, however, it was like this before, then it changes towards a black colour as a consequence of overheating. Hence Hippocrates wrote as follows concerning pleurisy: 'It is neces-

K293 sary to cut the inner vein at the elbow and not shrink from withdrawing a large quantity, until it flows much redder or yellower, or becomes livid instead of clear and red; for either may happen.'[63] He establishes the change appearing in the blood as a sign that some from the inflamed part has been received into the vein that has been opened. It is not, however, always desirable to await this; there are times when one ought to stop earlier, for two reasons: either because of the weakness of the faculties or because of the malignancy of the inflammation. Sometimes the vein lets nothing out, being strongly constricted. But if the faculties do not appear to have been dissolved by the evacuation – and you can tell[64] this by feeling the pulse – it is appropriate to await the change, as long as the person phlebotomised is in the prime of life, and particularly if the ambient air is temperate. These are the two things that are chiefly responsible for the uncertainty about the amount of the evacuation: what the nature of the patient is, since we are unable to determine it exactly, and what sort of temperament of the ambient air will prevail after the phlebotomy. Whenever the feverish heat spreads much of the blood

K294 abroad, and the patient is inadequately fed, it must be that the power of the blood to nourish him quickly becomes inadequate, with the result that his faculties are dissolved. The nourishment is used up both because of the temperament of the patient, which is damp and hot, as that of children also is, and because of the air that surrounds him in a

---

[62] Reading ἀψευδεῖ with La and K's translator.   [63] L 2, 272.

[64] Reading εἰδῇς with the translators of K and Ju; all the MSS have the same reading as K.

hot region and the summer season.[65] For this reason, therefore, we remove less than the plethos would otherwise demand at their time of life, in the case of children; we are guided by the habit of body in the case of soft-fleshed and fair patients like the Celts; and we take the time of year into consideration, during the dog days. It is the same with regions and states of the weather. On the other hand, as mentioned earlier in the case of the opposite conditions – that is, cold seasons and regions – we are on our guard against copious evacuations because of the consequent chilling. Hence we cannot lay down in black and white a fixed amount to be removed in each of the conditions mentioned. I have known myself remove as much as six pounds[66] of blood from some patients, extinguishing the fever forthwith and doing the faculties no harm; yet in others one and a half could not be taken without some slight injury to the faculties, and if two had been taken from these patients, the gravest damage would have resulted. Thus I know that I have sometimes removed as little as one pound with benefit, and sometimes even less, from a vein in the K295 elbow, ham or ankle, as I have also done from the veins at the greater canthi of the eyes or under the tongue. There is not usually a notable flow; nor is there if one cuts a vein in the foot or in the finger-tips, as those do who intend to treat the spleen by opening a vein alongside the second of the small fingers. More of this later.

15. If I were to write everything that has been said on this subject by doctors, I should need a large book, and would fill it to capacity. But, just as I have done with the other matters that have been explained up to this point in the argument, I have merely reminded you of my own opinion, since you have seen it confirmed in practice. I shall do the same now, basing my argument on things that can be clearly seen every day in clinical practice, which Hippocrates, who observed them carefully, was the first to describe.[67] The one chief point of them is that those conditions that bleed *kat' ixin* bring the greatest help to the sick. K296 That *kat' ixin* means 'on the same side as the lesion' is generally agreed; it is well known that the words *kat' ixin* are often used in this sense.

---

[65] Climate is far more important in Galen's system than it is today. Transpiration is increased when the weather is hot; thus one should remove less blood in the season of summer and in hot regions, such as Egypt.

[66] Six Roman pounds is about two litres of blood. See nn. 58 and 59 above.

[67] Bleeding from the left nostril brings relief when the spleen is enlarged (L 5, 86, 94) but haemorrhages from the unaffected side (e.g. from the right nostril in splenomegaly) are harmful (L 5, 554, 654). There are several references in *Epidemics* IV to haemorrhages taking place on the left in affections of the spleen, but no comment on whether they did good; they are noted as if a recognised occurrence (L 5, 144–97). In *Epidemics* VI doubt is expressed whether the rule applies to conditions moving from above downwards, or only in the opposite direction, though the passage is obscure (L 5, 278–80). There is a similar passage in *Epidemics* II (L 5, 110–12).

Those, however, that bleed on the opposite side do not help at all, and sometimes even do harm by dissolving the faculties without alleviating the disease. A haemorrhage from the right nostril confers no benefit on an enlarged spleen, nor does one from the left nostril benefit the liver; but revulsion, in those submitted to this treatment, shows quick and obvious benefit when performed on the affected side, whereas on the opposite side it does not. When the right nostril is bleeding, a cupping glass applied to the right hypochondrium brings a quick and evident end to the haemorrhage, as does one on the left in a patient bleeding from the left nostril. When you are phlebotomising to achieve revulsion, you will soon see clear benefit from bleedings on the affected side; if you were to cut on the opposite side, however, it would be of no use.[68]

16. So also when the spleen is affected, incision of the vein in the ring finger of the left hand is of benefit, just as it would be if you were K297 to cut the inner vein at the elbow; for evacuation of blood from the left hand helps a disordered spleen considerably. It is better, however, not to let out the appropriate amount at one operation, but to spread it over two days. Indeed I cannot tell why physicians have neglected to phlebotomise patients with diseases of the spleen; for myself, I have always known great benefit to follow, even if one were to evacuate only one pound. One should, however, decide the amount of the evacuation from the aforementioned indications. In pleuritic patients, phlebotomy on the same side as the affected rib has often shown the clearest benefit, while if it is on the opposite side, the benefits are either quite indefinite or are seen only after some time has elapsed. Phlebotomy on the affected side has often checked, within an hour, the severest pains in the eye, when the vein known as the humeral is cut. It is better, and might be tried in all diseases, after moderate amounts of blood have been let, to perform the procedure called epaphairesis, sometimes on the same day when this is practicable, and sometimes on the following one, except when, as previously men-K298 tioned, we intend to undertake evacuation to loss of consciousness. When the eyes are affected, cutting the vein called the humeral, or the one branching from it at the elbow, quickly brings clear benefit. When, on the other hand, the ribs, lung, diaphragm, spleen or liver and stomach are involved, the vein is the one that passes through the armpit to arrive at the elbow joint; cut this, particularly the inner vein, or failing that the vein branching from it towards the flexure of the joint. You know, I suppose, that the said vein splits off from the

---

[68] The question of letting blood from the side of the body on which the lesion is situated is discussed in Chapter 8 below, pp. 140–4.

humeral vein a little further back, and is connected with it. There are these three ways of performing phlebotomy at the elbow: inner, outer, and middle.[69] The inner is helpful for those who suffer from conditions of the lower part of the neck; the outer where parts above this, or the face or head, are involved. The middle site sometimes has both the branching veins extending to the end of the arm, and uniting there, and sometimes running to unite quickly with each other at the bend of the elbow. Sometimes one of them is prominent, the other indistinct. When, therefore, the vein that ought to be used for the K299 parts affected is indistinct, you may have recourse to one of the middle ones; try, for preference, to cut the one that branches from the proper vein. At times, again, there is no objection to opening veins lower than the elbow joint, in the forearm, when those at the elbow are not prominent; here again use those on the affected side. Used in this way, phlebotomies on the side of the affected parts sometimes bring quick and obvious benefit, so as frequently to astonish both the patients themselves and their families.

17. I remember once being sent for by a certain rich man living in a suburb of Rome to see one of his stewards, who was, to quote his own words, in danger of going blind; he was in great pain and had suffered this for nearly twenty days. There was an Erasistratean physician who attended the rich man's household, who made a practice of abstaining from phlebotomy at all times. On examination I found that the patient was young and full-blooded, and did not yet have any ulceration of the eyes, although the inflammation was extremely severe, with K300 discharge and thickening of both eyelids; he already had some rough patches on one, as a result of which his vision was dimmed, the pain made still worse, and the inflammation and discharge were exacerbated. When I had seen this for myself, and acquainted myself with the whole course of treatment that the physician had undertaken, I said that I[70] was not able to come to the suburb frequently, and that I

---

[69] See below, Chapter 8, pp. 140–1, for Galen's nomenclature and anatomy. The humeral vein is the modern cephalic; this is his outer vein at the elbow. The inner is the basilic, and the middle one is the median cubital vein.

[70] This is the only likely meaning, and is that of Kühn's Latin, Fu, Ju and Cobet (*Mnemosyne* n.s. 13 (1885) 1) I am indebted to Dr Nutton for bringing him to my attention. It requires the reading αὐτὸς μὲν οὐκ ἔφην. All the MSS, however, have the same text as K's Greek, which can only mean 'he said that he [i.e. some person other than the speaker] could not come'. By emending ἔφη to ἔφην we get the meaning 'I said that he [i.e. the Erasistratean] could not come', and this is the reading of Ald, which however spoils its record by repeating ἔφην at line 10, where the reading can only be ἔφη. Here we must suppose that the Erasistratean was present, and that Galen (tactfully, for once) was saying 'Of course a busy consultant like you can't be always rushing off to the suburbs'. There is nothing else in the account to suggest that he was there.

would need to see the patient at short intervals until the third day; 'So give him to me', I said, 'for these three days.' 'I'll agree to that thankfully', he replied, 'take the man to your house at once.' He must have arrived, I suppose, about the fifth hour, and was at once deprived[71] of three pounds of blood[72] at the first bleeding, followed by a further pound at the ninth hour. Much relieved[73] by these evacuations, he was rubbed the next day with one of the soft collyria mixed with wine, as we usually do in such cases, by interposition[74] of the rounded end of a probe[75] under thé eyelids. This was done first thing

K301 in the morning, then at the fourth hour, and again at the ninth. After these anointings he bathed about sunset, and the next day, after his eyelids had been everted, he was rubbed twice with soft collyrium mixed into a far larger amount of wine, and after this he bathed at evening. Early the next day he met the rich man at a certain place where they usually get out of their carriages,[76] and saluted him[77] with his eyes open and free from inflammation and discharge – the same man who, two days earlier, had been unable to open his eyelids because of the discharge and the pain. The thing seemed almost to have taken place by some kind of magic, causing the rich man to exclaim in astonishment at the rapidity of the cure, and all those with him to raise a shout in the same way, not because I had done something great, but at the comparison between what I had done and the efforts of his household physician who had caused such grave harm through his fear of phlebotomy. The patient had needed the crusts and roughnesses to be wiped off his eyelids, which could not be

K302 done without using a corrosive drug; and he could not stand such a drug unless he had first been evacuated. I have often said, and proved, that all biting drugs, to whatever parts they are applied, attract a flow of humours and cause inflammation if the whole body is not empty and completely free from residues. The rich man then enquired what magical treatment had taken place, and when he had heard everything that had been done, he gave the Erasistratean physician the title of 'Haemophobe' from that time on. The account includes a demonstration, both of the need to phlebotomise patients with such conditions, which I have not considered in the present work, and of the need to phlebotomise on the same side as the affected

---

[71] Reading ἀφῃρέθη with Cobet (p. 2).   [72] About a litre.
[73] Reading ἀνακύψας with La.
[74] Reading καθ' ὑποβολὴν with La, A and U. LSJ gives the authority of Oribasius for the meaning of interposition or anointing under the eyelid. Collyrium is an eye-salve.
[75] Reading μηλης with M. See also K x, 202.
[76] This account casts an interesting light on transport arrangements in second-century Rome.
[77] Reading αὐτον with La.

parts, and to cut the humeral veins in lesions of the parts above the level of the chest.

18. Just as the abovementioned parts are benefited, as I have said, by phlebotomies performed at the elbow, in the same way those parts that are lower down than these are helped by venesections at the hams and ankles. Those that are lower than the aforesaid parts are the parts in the region of the hip, bladder and uterus. The kidneys have a double significance, situated as they are below the parts first men- K303 tioned, but above these mentioned second, and hence they sometimes yield to phlebotomies at the elbow, when there is recent inflammation and a plethos of blood. In patients with the condition they specifically call nephritis, you should cut the vein in the ham, or the veins alongside the ankles. Inflammatory conditions of the uterus are benefited even more than those of the kidneys by the veins in the legs being cut. There is an additional difficulty with evacuations at the elbow; for they check the menstrual purgations, diverting the blood towards the upper parts of the body. By evacuations from the legs, however, it is possible not only to revulse, but also to urge on the menses. When you wish to achieve this at the time when the woman's period is due, start about three or four days in advance by cutting a vein or scarifying the malleoli of one leg, and draw off a little blood; then on the next day evacuate in the same way from the other leg, at the same time prescribing a reducing diet for the days on which you evacuate thus, and in the four or five days preceding them. I have written a special work on the reducing diet. But even in women who K304 are not on this diet, mint and pennyroyal bring on an abundant menstrual flow. Administer them to the women boiled in melicratum, dry, chopped up, and passed through a fine sieve, and then again rubbed to make them as fine as dust, and sprinkled on melicratum. The best time for the draught is after the bath, when the women have been wrapped in bandages. These are drugs of moderate strength; more powerful are savin and dittany, which are used in the same way as the drugs previously mentioned. Also to be administered at this time is the preparation commonly known as bitter, consisting of a hundred drachms of aloes mixed with six of each of the other drugs. It is best when the patient takes cinnamon. These things deserve mention in passing; yet they are not of secondary importance, since in combination with the evacuations from the legs they promote the flow of blood from the uterus when the ankles have been scarified or a vein opened in the heel or the ham. I have known diseases of the hip cured in one day by an evacuation through the legs; such of them, that is, as have not arisen as a result of cold, but through blood having collected K305 in the veins in the ischial region. Hence phlebotomy from the ham is more effective than from the ankles in patients thus affected, and scarification brings them no obvious benefit.

19. To put it briefly, incipient inflammations ought to be evacuated revulsively, but chronic ones, where possible, through the affected parts, or failing this through those nearest to them. This is because in those that are starting, one should turn back the fluxion that is descending on them, while in those that have become chronic one should evacuate only the material that has already become fixed[78] in the affected part. This is best let out through the veins that are connected with those[79] in the part concerned. Experience also bears out this conclusion. Parts in the region of the throat and trachea which are much inflamed are greatly benefited at the beginning by venesection at the elbow, but after the beginning by letting blood from the tongue; both the veins in it are cut. So too cutting the vein alongside the greater canthus is good for the crusts on the eyes that remain after K306 inflammations. Similarly when a vein in the forehead is cut, heaviness of the head and pains that have become chronic as a result of plethos are usually noticeably relieved; but when they are starting, or are at their height, revulsion at the neck by means of a cupping glass relieves them, sometimes by itself, sometimes when used in combination with scarifications. The whole body should be evacuated in advance. In the same way pains in the back of the head, whether incipient or already established, are relieved by cutting the vein in the forehead. When fluxions are beginning, one should preferably effect revulsion in combination with evacuation; but when, for instance, inflammatory conditions have gone on to induration, evacuate through the affected parts, or adjacent ones. In bodies of which no part is yet affected, but we are evacuating prophylactically at the beginning of spring – in these, if the patient is liable to be seized with feverish diseases in the summer season, our aim is to evacuate their excess, and any part of the body is equally good for the removal of the blood. This applies also if K307 the patient is arthritic in all his joints. But in those who have some part particularly affected and have not undergone prophylactic evacuation, one should not make the evacuation from any part indiscriminately, but it should be done as in those who have already begun to sicken. Hence one should evacuate gouty patients from the elbow, but epileptics and scotomatics preferably from the legs.[80] If you have

---

[78] Reading ἐνσφηνουμένον, as K's Latin (infixum) suggests.

[79] Reading ταις with La.

[80] I.e. open a vein remote from the affected parts, the legs and brain respectively, to direct the fluxions away from them.

recourse to phlebotomy because of suppression of a haemorrhoid, and wish to restrain the bleeding further, you should cut the veins in the arms; but to urge it on, those in the legs. When the menses are suppressed, however, those in the legs are invariably used. This is because the situation where the menstrual purgation is concerned is not the same as with haemorrhoids, where some people may wish to be relieved of such an evacuation while others are glad to retain it. The evacuation from haemorrhoids is in danger of reaching such an immoderate degree as to kill the patient forthwith, or to render him grossly hydropic or cachectic; but nothing of the sort happens with the evacuations from the uterus, as long as they are according to nature. It sometimes happens, however, that even the uterus bleeds from an erosion, and in these patients the aim of treatment is not the same; we K308 do not wish the blood to flow as it does in the menses, but at all costs to stanch it. This rule applies to all those coming to phlebotomy at the beginning of spring; if they have some particularly weak part to which the accumulated plethos extends,[81] evacuate revulsively; where, however, there is no part thus affected, one may let blood from any part one chooses, except in the case of suppression of haemorrhoids or of the menses, as laid down a little earlier.[82]

20. The matter now under consideration has been dealt with virtually throughout the previous account; it is as well, however, to go through everything again now, on the one hand to collect into one passage everything previously said, and on the other to draw the distinctions that have not been drawn. It should be taken as a general rule that one ought not to consider in the first place a time limit of so many days for phlebotomy, as some have written, and some have most ridiculously set at the paroxysm on the third day, when, as they say, we could already have some knowledge of the sort of disease we have to deal with in its variety and character, and its entire nature. K309 Others again lay down the fourth day as the utmost limit for phlebotomy, and within this period they agree in phlebotomising whenever they choose in the intervals between paroxysms. Still others make haste to let blood on whatever days they may define the need for its removal, provided that it is still moving from one part to another, and has not yet become firmly installed in some part that has received the excess. They consider only one factor, whether some corruption of the food digested in the belly may have occurred, or some delay in

---

[81] La appears to omit the word διήχει, though the MS is in bad condition here. It is certainly absent in A, U and M.

[82] A, U and M end the work here and go on to another work of Galen, *On Theriac against Pamphilianus.*

digestion, or, again, whether the food may have been held up in it. Accordingly, when they say that it is necessary to make haste in the case of patients who need evacuation – except, presumably, when there is need for the food and the half-digested juices in the first veins to be digested – they speak very correctly, and are to be trusted. Since, however, we are often called to attend someone only after five or six days have elapsed since the onset, it would be proper to bleed him even though the first opportunity for using the remedy has been missed. For on whatever day you observe the indications[83] for

K310 phlebotomy in the patient, on that day you will apply the remedy, even if it is the twentieth day from the onset. And what are the indications? The disease severe; strength of the faculties; except in the stage of childhood, and when the ambient air is very hot. Since, in most diseases, the patient's strength will already have been diminished with the passage of time, the opportunity for phlebotomy is lost because of the number[84] of days that have elapsed; this, however, is not a primary[85] effect, but is due to the intervention of another factor, namely the antecedent dissolution of the faculties. Hence, if even on the second day after the onset the powers should appear to be dissolved, we shall refrain from phlebotomy.

21. Again, I think it is clear that on the particular day on which we are to phlebotomise we ought to watch out for the abatement of the fever; but this is not clear to some people, the sort who order phlebotomy only at daybreak, or up to the fifth and sixth hour at the latest. If, however, anyone calls to mind what has been said pre-

K311 viously in the whole of this work, he will make no such mistake, but will phlebotomise at any hour of the day and throughout the night, taking as his indication the decline in the individual paroxysms in patients with fever, and the need for the remedy – because of ophthalmia or some other such condition – in those without it; not the abatement, seeing that fever is totally absent in these, but the severity of the pain or inflammation or the patient's whole condition, in which there is need for phlebotomy. But where nothing of this kind either urges or forbids us, it is best to phlebotomise at daybreak, not immediately after patients have risen from sleep, but after they have been awake for about an hour, and it is said that it is better for some patients to bathe, and if they do, that some of them should take a walk before doing so. In the case of those in whom we have recourse to

---

[83] Here, as in several other places, I have rendered σκοπός by 'indication', since the meaning seems unmistakable.

[84] Reading πρὸς τοῦ πλήθους. La reads ἀναιρεῖται ὡς πληθει.   [85] Reading πρῶτον.

phlebotomy at the beginning of spring, I have known myself phlebotomise some, in expectation of fever, even after they have finished some of their customary tasks, whether in the schools, the workshops, the forum or the home. As for the time for epaphairesis, in those patients in whom we decide simply to evacuate, this should take place on the same day; but for those who are revulsed,[86] it is better that it K312 should be done on two successive days. You should monitor the strength of the patient in all such cases, by feeling his pulse, since some patients are sensitive where strength is concerned, so that they cannot bear copious evacuation. In such cases, the patient should be allowed to recover[87] on the first day, and epaphairesis should be performed on the second.

22. I have shown elsewhere that the ancients applied the term vein to arteries as well, and this was agreed by others before us. Because of this, and because the subject-matter would be similar, and in the interests of brevity of expression, I thought it better not to write a separate book about arteriotomy, but to make this addendum to the work on phlebotomy, in that part where I consider which veins one should cut when particular parts are affected. For just as I have shown how certain veins correspond to certain parts, so also the practice is for physicians to cut the arteries in the temples and those behind the ears; those in the temples in the case of fluxions of the eyes, when these are hot and spirituous, and those behind the ears chiefly in scotomatics K313 and patients who suffer from chronic hot and spirituous[88] pains in the head. Some have already used arteriotomy behind the ears for other long-established conditions in the region of the head.[89] But they have not used it where another part is affected, although many parts in fact require it more than they do phlebotomy; since when hot and spirituous blood causes trouble through being crowded into the arteries, there is need for the arteries common to the affected parts to be cut. Since, however, the arteries are hard to stanch, doctors do not dare to cut them, and where some, while performing phlebotomy, have inadvertently wounded an artery, they have had difficulty in stopping the haemorrhage. When they do the best they can, an aneurysm develops in the incision scar.

---

[86] K's Greek omits a line, which is translated in his Latin version. La reads ἐφ᾽ ὧν μεν ἁπλῶς κενῶσαι βουλομεθα, και κατα την αὐτην ἡμεραν γινεσθω ἐφ᾽ ὧν δε ἀντισπασεται κἀν δυο ταις ἐφεξῆς ἡμεραις γενεται βελτιον ἐστι . . .

[87] Reading ἀνακτησάμενον with La.

[88] Spirituous because the arteries, in Galen's system, contain pneuma (spiritus) as well as blood. It is not clear what the characteristics of a spirituous pain are.

[89] Aretaeus performed arteriotomy in front of and behind the ears in epilepsy (vii.4.2).

23. I have, however, also known patients to die because of the artery that underlies the inner vein at the elbow; some quickly, K314 because of the tourniquet that was put round when the doctors wished to check the haemorrhage, with resulting gangrene, while others expired later while undergoing surgery for their aneurysms; for in the course of this operation it is necessary to tie off the vessel with a ligature. For these reasons doctors avoid the arteries that are notable for their size, while they also shun the small ones as being unable to effect anything of any importance. Nevertheless I have often seen these bring no small benefit, and at the same time to cicatrise completely without an aneurysm. Even if the artery is larger, however, it will also cicatrise without an aneurysm if it is cut completely through, and this procedure also often prevents the danger of haemorrhage. It can be clearly seen that the whole artery is cut[90] obliquely right through its whole substance, and the two parts are drawn up away from each other, the one above the site, the other below it. This also happens with veins, but only to a moderate degree, and always far more with arteries than with veins. I shall now tell you how I got the inspiration to have recourse to arteriotomy. Urged on by certain K315 dreams I had, two of which were particularly vivid, I went for the artery in the space between the index finger and thumb of the right hand, and allowed the blood to flow until it stopped of its own accord, as the dream commanded. Not quite a pound escaped. Forthwith a long-standing pain was relieved which had oppressed chiefly the part where the liver meets the diaphragm. This happened to me in my youth. And a worshipper of the god in Pergamon was relieved of a chronic pain in the side by an arteriotomy performed at the extremity of the hand; he also came upon this as the result of a dream. In another patient who had suffered a laceration of an artery in the ankle, the flow of blood did not cease until I was called and cut the entire artery through, after which I used a preparation made from aloes, frankincense and white of egg compounded with hare's fur,[91] and the wound healed without an aneurysm by the mouth of the artery becoming surrounded with flesh. The patient, who had suffered for four years from a good deal of pain in the hip, at last recovered from it. These experiences persuaded me often to open K316 arteries in the extremities of the limbs, and indeed in the head too, in the case of all pains that seemed to have their origin from a hot and spirituous quality, and particularly in the membranes.[92] In these, the

---

[90] Reading διεκόπη.
[91] The fur would have provided a framework for a clot to form on.
[92] Presumably the peritoneum and pleura.

pain has a pricking quality and spreads out gently, since the pricking sensation is located in one part as if this were the centre of the affected region, and the whole part[93] round this centre has a sensation of tension.

[93] Reading μοριου with La. K has μυός, 'muscle', which makes less good sense.

CHAPTER 5

Development of Galen's views and methods as shown in the three works

The dating of the three works will be considered later, but it is clear that the first work, the *De Venae Sectione adversus Erasistratum*, was composed soon after Galen's first arrival in Rome; it is representative, therefore, of his youthful opinions.[1] There is nothing in this work to suggest that Galen, at that stage of his life, considered using any evacuant remedy other than phlebotomy at the onset of the patient's illness. He agrees with Erasistratus that it is necessary to empty the plethos; the only question is by what means it should be evacuated. 'I have always thought that once evacuation has been agreed on, the easiest and most prompt remedy is to open a vein, since in this way the inflammatory matters, and these alone, are evacuated as quickly as possible.'[2] All patients with plethos, he says, are most quickly and effectively treated by opening the veins; although Galen mentions alternative remedies used by Erasistratus, there is no indication that he uses any of them himself in these circumstances.[3] Not only the physicians of the rationalist sect, but also the empiricists, all use venesection; even Asclepiades, who condemned all the dogmas of his predecessors and described the Hippocratic methods as an exercise in death.[4] It is in use in most diseases and the most acute, and Hippocrates himself, 'whom we regard as the leader of all the distinguished men in the profession, and the other men of old clearly did use it'.[5] The ancients, in Galen's opinion, thought it nothing less than the most effective of all remedies.[6] Purgatives and other evacuant drugs are dangerous because once they have been administered their action cannot be stopped; the flow of blood, on the other hand, can be

---

[1] He describes the circumstances in which it was dictated in his second work on venesection (K xi, 193–5; see above, pp. 41–2) and in K xix, 13–14. Johannes Ilberg, 'Ueber die Schriftstellerei des Klaudios Galenos', *Rh. Mus.* 44 (1889) 207–39 (i); 47 (1892) 489–514 (ii); 51 (1896) 165–96 (iii); 52 (1897) 591–623 (iv) dates Galen's first sojourn in Rome between 164 and 168 (i, 228). K. Bardong ('Beiträge zur Hippokrates- und Galenforschung', *Nachr. Akad. Gött. Phil. Hist. Kl.* 7 (1942) 577–640 (p. 633) places it at 162 to 166. V. Nutton ('The chronology of Galen's early career', *Class. Quart.* 23 (1973) 158–71) argues convincingly that he arrived in August, September or October 162 and left in August 166; he returned in 169.

[2] K xi, 156.　　[3] K xi, 178–9.　　[4] K xi, 163.　　[5] K xi, 150.　　[6] K xi, 147–8.

terminated at will.[7] Erasistratus, however, pins his faith on the exhausting remedy of starving his patients to death.[8] Galen criticises this on the grounds that fasting, not being a thing that exists in itself, but only a deprivation of an existing thing, cannot be an evacuant remedy.[9] Starvation alone is useless; it can, however, be used in combination with other remedies, though even here the damage it does outweighs the advantages of the evacuation.[10] Erasistratus is pitiably stupid; he uses nothing but starvation at the onset of the disease. 'I do not open a vein' he says, 'so that the patient may be strong enough to bear the fasting imposed because of the inflammation.' But why, asks Galen, does he starve the patient with inflammation at all? and Galen makes him reply that it is to empty the veins. Why then, says Galen, did he not empty the veins by opening them? A thing that neither Hippocrates nor Diocles neglected he considers useless, namely to open the veins; he uses starvation and nothing else as a remedy. So, when he needs an evacuant remedy he arrives at the weakest of them all, neglecting the most effective ones and those that can most quickly lead to the desired effect.[11] Erasistratus, says Galen, praises nature but does not emulate her. She cures many diseases by means of naturally occurring haemorrhages, but Erasistratus will not let blood in a single one.[12] Galen contemplates the works of nature and bases his treatment on them; but as for Erasistratus, he is either completely stupid or little versed in the operations of nature. He is guilty either way; either he knows nothing, or he does not put what he knows into effect. He must have written these things shut up in some house, without ever examining a patient; this is evidently why he ignores the works of nature. He is always admiring her and never imitating her, which makes him unintelligent in the last degree.[13] Erasistratus does not even keep to the rules of correct writing; he should first expound the operations of nature and then draw conclusions; one should learn from nature's successes and apply her methods in cases where she needs assistance. But Erasistratus neglected to examine patients; he stayed at home and wrote down mere opinions. He might still have been a good physician, however, if he had only read Hippocrates;[14] 'but you seem to me to be exceptionally stupid because of your feud with Hippocrates'. Opposites are cured by their opposites; this is the doctrine of all men, not only of the father of medicine. Even laymen know that patients who are suffocating with angina or peripneumonia must be venesected; irrational brutes provoke vomiting and give themselves enemas; but

---

[7] K xi, 172–3.   [8] K xi, 182.   [9] K xi, 183–5.   [10] K xi, 186.   [11] K xi, 176–8.
[12] K xi, 158.   [13] K xi, 158–9.   [14] K xi, 159–60.

Erasistratus is less intelligent even than the cranes.[15] He is like blind men, who, when a smooth, straight and wide road lies before them, go instead by a narrow, rough and long detour; he considers only whether it leads him to his destination, and not whether it gets there quickly or without trouble. The wise Erasistratus, says Galen, sees fit to neglect so great a remedy, which many of the Hippocratic physicians thought worthy of application. 'But Hippocrates did not take this view of phlebotomy, O Erasistratus, and he was in no way a worse physician than you are.'[16] The Erasistratean physicians of Galen's time are even worse than their master; they are ignorant men, who in addition to raving about things that have no rational basis, know nothing about the things they praise. They stand in awe of the words of Erasistratus, and assume his name, calling themselves Erasistrateans, but they are so ignorant of them that they expound everything except his opinion.

So, concerning phlebotomy, they utter such egregious and portentous absurdities as to make one stand amazed, not only at their ignorance, but at their shamelessness as well ... Do you wish me, then, to pay attention to those people who talk nonsense on behalf of Erasistratus, when I have the very words of Erasistratus to consult? ... I need not go back to the raving Erasistratus to tell me why he said that food should not be given to patients suffering from inflammation; I have Erasistratus himself expounding it.[17]

But if Erasistratus would open his ears, or, better still, his mind, Galen could teach him something.[18]

The second work (*De Venae Sectione adversus Erasistrateos Romae Degentes*) dates from Galen's second period in Rome, and shows a most remarkable change of attitude. At certain times and for certain indications we should use fasting, at others phlebotomy, he says,[19] though fasting should not be used after venesection.[20] Phlebotomy ought to be avoided in those patients who are to be fasted, since it is not possible to use both remedies in the same patient.[21] It is not necessary, Galen now holds, to prohibit venesection entirely, nor on the other hand to hold that it is called for in all those for whom Erasistratus prescribed starvation, as the Erasistrateans of his time maintain.[22] These latter-day disciples of Erasistratus neglect the factors that should sometimes restrain them from phlebotomy.[23] They think venesection is necessary at every onset of fever;[24] as far as can be ascertained from Galen's first work, this was his own opinion in his youth, but he certainly does not hold it now. He says of the new generation of self-styled Erasistrateans:

[15] K xi, 167–9.   [16] K xi, 157.   [17] K xi, 174–6.   [18] K xi, 169.   [19] K xi, 224.
[20] K xi, 199, 204.   [21] K xi, 247.   [22] K xi, 195.   [23] K xi, 196.   [24] K xi, 223.

But the fact that the new physicians have recourse to the remedy without knowing anything about the amount of blood that should be let and the veins that should be cut will do the greatest harm to patients, as I said right at the beginning. It would be better for them to renounce phlebotomy altogether than to use the remedy without paying attention to such matters. More patients have been lost in this way than have died at the hands of those who did not use phlebotomy. The old practitioners of those days who never used phlebotomy at all employed other evacuant remedies which could achieve, although in a longer time, the same effect as phlebotomy, except where, because of the vital nature of the affected part or the excess of the plethos, the patient forestalled them by expiring. Today's doctors, however, who think that every onset of fever demands phlebotomy, do no inconsiderable harm to the sick.[25]

As for Erasistratus himself, he recommends starvation and mistakenly does away with venesection, yet he is less at fault than those who suppose that all patients who need starvation should forthwith be venesected.[26] Galen must make his recantation to those Erasistrateans whom he has persuaded, with his first work, to use venesection, exhorting them to spend as long as they like fighting about words, but to have mercy on their patients,[27] and persuading those who are bleeding rashly that it would be better not to bleed at all.[28]

In this book Erasistratus comes in for very little criticism; he is even described, though not by Galen, as an excellent physician.[29] Although Galen gently makes fun of his prolixity in describing the preparation of barley-cake or the cooking of chicory,[30] there are none of the abusive remarks about him in the second book that are such a notable feature of the first. The same cannot be said of his followers; they lie four times over,[31] and are abusive and stupid,[32] making rash pronouncements about things of which they know nothing.[33] In spite of this, the tone of the second work is altogether much less venomous than that of the first. This, no doubt, is partly because the first book is a verbatim record of an emotional public meeting; even allowing for this, however, the second is far milder.

The third work (*De Curandi Ratione per Venae Sectionem*) is not controversial at all, being concerned chiefly with pathology and methods of treatment, and will not be considered in detail. It observes again that venesection is not always necessary in plethoric patients;[34] some patients have a condition that requires the remedy, but are unable to bear it.[35] Nothing derogatory is said about Erasistratus, but his disciples are evidently still at their tricks; they still believe that

[25] K xi, 223. [26] K xi, 247–8. [27] K xi, 195. [28] K xi, 224. [29] K xi, 210.
[30] K xi, 214–15. [31] K xi, 236. [32] K xi, 228–9. [33] K xi, 221–2.
[34] K xi, 261. [35] K xi, 250.

venesection should be used in all those patients for whom their master would have used fasting at the onset of the illness. It would be a great evil, says Galen, if this pernicious doctrine were to spread. It is better that the Erasistrateans should believe that their master never used venesection than that they should employ it indiscriminately.[36]

What is the reason for this remarkable change of front? A clue can be found in a remark of Galen's in the second book, concerning the effects of his first work.

The work was composed in a manner not befitting a book but rather a lecture room, at the request of my friend that it should be dictated just as it had been spoken; but even such as it was, and having many deficiencies compared with the ideal, it nevertheless seemed to achieve somewhat more than I expected. For all those who now call themselves Erasistrateans have come round to the opposite opinion, and are lining up all and sundry to be phlebotomised, not only patients like those mentioned earlier, but also those who are in any way feverish.[37]

In doing this, however, they did not renounce their allegiance to Erasistratus; they merely announced that he had used phlebotomy after all, but had neglected to mention it because it was self-evident.[38] Galen goes to the most tedious lengths to demolish this argument in the second book, which opens with a lively account of events at the time of his first arrival in Rome, and continues with an intolerably repetitive proof that Erasistratus was never a venesectionist. The first two works amply confirm Galen's repeated assertions that the Erasistrateans of his time were an ignorant lot; what is remarkable, however, is the obvious, and to Galen wholly unexpected, success of his campaign to convert them. His methods, as described in the second book, were to say the least tactless. 'Before this' he says, 'I had been afraid to argue with the doctors, since I guessed what they would say to avoid having to use phlebotomy; but now, since it seemed obvious to everyone that the woman had been saved at the moment when the evacuation of blood took place, I reminded them of those who had died, pointing out that if someone had phlebotomised them they might perhaps have been saved.'[39] His colleague Teuthras,

a fellow-citizen and schoolfellow of mine – he was exceedingly frank in his ways – said: 'You will never influence these men; they are too stupid to remember the patients who were killed by Erasistratus. For what other reason did the patients they are citing now come to die, if not that the remedy of phlebotomy was omitted? and why else did the patients die who were prevented by these men from being evacuated in good time?' and he

---

[36] K xi, 254.   [37] K xi, 194–5.   [38] K xi, 196–7.   [39] K xi, 191.

enumerated them all in order, together with the conditions they had, which I mentioned a little earlier. Then he smiled and threw up his hands, and drawing me after him forcibly he led me away from the doctors. The next day he brought out the books of Erasistratus on divisions and read them to all the philosophers, with the aim of showing that the girl from Chios and Criton had died because of Erasistratus, and of trying to provoke the senior physicians to debate. But they did not arrive, thinking it beneath their dignity to contend with a youth. At that time the custom had somehow sprung up of speaking in public each day on questions that were put forward, and someone posed the question whether Erasistratus had been right in not using phlebotomy. I dealt in detail with this question, which seemed to those listening at the time a very good one; this was the reason why Teuthras also urged me to dictate what I had said to a boy whom he would send. He said he was particularly anxious to have it since he was planning to visit Ionia and was on the point of leaving. I was accordingly persuaded by my companion and dictated the speech. It so happened that the book leaked out to many people; it was not deliberately spread abroad by him.[40]

Further interesting details of this meeting appear in a late work of Galen's, the tract *On His Own Books*. Galen's chief adversary at the gathering was a certain Martialius, an Erasistratean physician whose two books on anatomy were held in high regard at the time. Galen says that he was somewhat spiteful and contentious, though more than seventy years old. On hearing of Galen's successful public lectures he asked one of his friends to what sect Galen belonged, and was told that he regarded as slaves those who adhered strictly to the teaching of any one man, even if he was Hippocrates.

And once, when I was speaking on the books of the old physicians, the work of Erasistratus on bringing up blood was publicly put before me, and when a pen had been stuck into it, according to the custom, it indicated that part of the book in which he deprecates venesection. I criticised him at length so that I might annoy Martialius, who claims to be an Erasistratean; and since my address was very well received, a certain friend of mine, who was irritated by Martialius, asked me to dictate my remarks to a shorthand writer whom he would send, so that when he left the city for his home he might be able to quote my observations against him when visiting patients. Then, I can't say how, when I came to Rome the second time, summoned by the Emperors, the man who had taken the book had died, and many people had got possession of it. It has been written in the contentious spirit of the period when I was holding public disputes; for you must know that I was still young, thirty-four years of age, when I did this. From that time I determined not to teach publicly any longer or to give demonstrations, having succeeded in my practice beyond my hopes.[41]

---

[40] K xi, 193–4.
[41] K xix, 14–15. For Galen's eclectic attitude with regard to the sects, see K viii, 143–4.

In Galen's second work on venesection he tells us that the friend who requested the work was Teuthras. Even at this early stage of his life Galen seems a little ashamed of it, for he says: 'It so happened that the book leaked out to many people; it was not deliberately spread abroad by him.[42] The work was composed in a manner not befitting a book but rather a lecture room ... and having many deficiencies compared with the ideal.'[43]

It seems clear that it was not so much this discussion, but the book, when it became generally available, that persuaded the Erasistratean physicians that venesection was a useful procedure. Whatever its cause, however, the change in the practice of the Erasistrateans was dramatic. Galen makes it clear that although they assumed the name of their master they were largely ignorant of his writings;[44] this, perhaps, made it easier for them to believe anything about him that the occasion demanded. Clearly the new conviction, that Erasistratus had been a venesectionist, was widespread among them at the time of his second work, since Galen goes to great lengths to refute it.

Some sort of chronology is necessary in any study of the development of Galen's ideas and methods, and an attempt must therefore be made to date the three works on venesection. Two of them present no difficulty. The first, he tells us himself, was dictated soon after his first arrival in Rome, which took place late in AD 162; it can perhaps be dated to spring 163.[45] The third is a late work, composed after the last books of the *De Methodo Medendi*, some thirty years after the first work on venesection.[46] The interesting question is the date of the second work, *De Venae Sectione adversus Erasistrateos Romae Degentes*, which shows a notable change of attitude from the first work. Over what period did this change take place?

Bardong lists the criteria that can be used to date Galen's works. They are: (1) References to works already in existence, provided these are not later additions to the text; such additions can sometimes be recognised because they can be removed without damage to Galen's train of thought, and repeated citations of a particular work are less likely to be later interpolations than isolated references are. It is known

[42] See n. 40 above. This sentence is translated by Kotrc (1970, p. 176): 'It turned out that the book was widely read having been circulated by Teuthras contrary to my intentions.' Although the Greek might bear this interpretation, the passage from *On His Own Books* makes it clear, I think, that the dissemination took place only after Teuthras' death. The Latin translator in Kühn, however, renders it 'non ex mea sententia', i.e. 'not according to my wishes'.

[43] K xi, 194–5. Galen perhaps makes his amends in his work *On the Opinions of Hippocrates and Plato*, where he says that the opinions of Erasistratus on many subjects, though in his opinion false, are not deserving of ridicule (K v, 714–15).

[44] K xi, 175.   [45] K xi, 194–5.   [46] Ilberg III, 195.

that Galen made interpolations in the course of subsequent editing or rewriting of his works, to say nothing of those made by others. It is thus difficult for the reader of today to use cross-references to determine the order of their composition. (2) The use of the future tense to speak of works not yet written. (3) References to historical events. (4) References by Galen to his own life, or to his medical or literary activity. Homer, however, has been known to nod; Galen, says Bardong, can be mistaken about his literary output, and certainly has been on occasion.[47] To these criteria of Bardong two others may be added: (5) Linguistic; but Ilberg thinks linguistic analysis of little value in dating Galen's works,[48] and Bardong does not use it at all. (6) Psychological: Galen's attitude to his profession and to his colleagues unquestionably changed as his life advanced, and it is conceivable that early or late works might be tentatively identified in this way, though it would be a hazardous undertaking.

How might these criteria be used in the problem before us? The second work on venesection is remarkable in containing no mention whatever of any other works of Galen except the first on venesection, so that the least help is available precisely where the most is needed. The only criteria that can be used are the third, fourth and sixth; even if linguistic criteria were of value, specialised techniques would be necessary to apply them. Ilberg's views on the dating of the second work will be considered first. He says:

The first work ... is the product of one of his public lectures, which, as previously shown, he delivered in his thirty-fourth year in Rome, and which is dedicated to his friend Teuthras. The second ... belongs to his second sojourn in Rome, as its opening words tell us. It is closely linked with the third ... as its conclusion shows. But it is clear that this connection was only established later. We learn more about their relationship in the introduction to the third book. 'In my view', says Galen himself, 'it was quite unnecessary to write a further book about bloodletting, since I had already dealt with the matter at length in two of my major works and in the two minor ones against Erasistratus and against the Erasistrateans in Rome. But because many friends in the profession repeatedly asked me to do so, I saw that I would have to bring myself to write the treatise now before you.' It is thus clear that at the time the second book was written there was no intention at all of writing the third; hence the whole concluding part of the second ... must have been added subsequently. There can be no doubt that a considerable time had elapsed before *On Treatment by Phlebotomy* followed the polemical works

---

[47] Bardong, pp. 604–6. There is some further recent discussion of these criteria, in connection with works of Galen not relevant to the present argument, in D. W. Peterson, 'Observations on the chronology of the Galenic corpus', *Bull. Hist. Med.* 51 (1977) 484–95.

[48] Ilberg I, 239.

against Erasistratus and his followers in Rome. How long this period was I cannot say, but it seems to me that the composition of the *On Treatment* took place only after the completion of the second part of the *De Methodo Medendi*, under Septimius Severus. Finally Galen decided to put all the three books on bloodletting together after brief editing, although thirty years must have separated the first and the last.[49]

There is no doubt that Ilberg's conclusion, that the end of the second work is a later addition by Galen, is correct. The promises made in it are fulfilled to the letter in the third work, and we may see the postscript as a connecting passage added by Galen during the 'flüchtige Redaktion' of the three works made towards the end of his life, perhaps just before he wrote *On His Own Books*, in which he lists the three together under the title 'Three concerning phlebotomy'.[50] The editing that they received, however, must indeed have been cursory, since Galen made no attempt to modify the tone of the first work, so different from that of the second and third, or to change his youthful opinions on the use of phlebotomy expressed in it. The relationship between the second and third works, therefore, is not as close as an uncritical reading of the end of the second might suggest. It remains to attempt a closer estimate of the date of the second work than Ilberg has achieved. He thinks that a considerable period elapsed between the second and third works, but cannot suggest how long it was, except that the third must be dated after the completion of the great *De Methodo Medendi*. This is clearly so; if we accept the dating of the last books of that work in the reign of Severus, AD 193 onwards, as both Ilberg and Bardong do, we can date the third work on vene-section in the last six years of Galen's life, assuming that he died about 200. This is also the absolute terminus for the second work on vene-section, since it is just conceivable that it is a late work, written just before the third and after the work on therapeutic method. It seems almost certain, however, that it is earlier than this work, in view of what Galen says in the third work:

It did not seem necessary, therefore, to me at any rate, to write anything more about phlebotomy, since the use of the remedy has been discussed in my book on therapeutic method, as well as in my books on health, and in the two I wrote, one against Erasistratus himself, the other against the Erasistrateans in Rome ... At the frequent request, however, of many friends in the profession, who seemed to me to have some aversion from reading *On Therapeutic Method*, I was compelled in the end to undertake the present work.[51]

---

[49] Ilberg III, 181–2 (translated).   [50] K XIX, 30–1.
[51] See translation, K 254, and Chapter 4, n. 5.

This strongly suggests that the mature fruit of his thought on vene-section was to be found in the *De Methodo Medendi*, where, were it not for the unmanageable proportions of the work, a reader might conveniently find all that he needed. It seems safe, therefore, to agree with Ilberg that some considerable time elapsed between the second and third works; the second was written before the last books of the *De Methodo Medendi*. On the very probable assumption that the latter part of that work took some considerable time to write,[52] the second work on venesection was finished before Severus came to the throne. The earlier terminus is quite definite; the work itself makes it clear that it was written during Galen's second sojourn in Rome, which began in 169. It could fall, therefore, anywhere in the two decades between 169 and 189 or thereabouts. Is there any internal evidence to place it more exactly in this period?

First, there has been a change in Galen's opinions and outlook. The first work shows them as they were in about 164; the second cannot be earlier than 169. Could they have changed as much as they did in five or six years? Allowing for the fact that the first work is avowedly polemical, and that Galen's real views, when he was not in an emotional situation, were probably more moderate, we must conclude that they could. The change in Galen's attitude, therefore, is not helpful in dating the second work.

In addition to the change in Galen, however, there is the change in the Erasistrateans. Previously they avoided phlebotomy; once conver-ted, like many converts they went to extremes. Galen makes a significant remark which suggests that it was not the public meeting soon after his arrival, but his book dictated after that meeting, that had this effect. 'The book leaked out to many people; it was not deliber-ately spread abroad by him ... It seemed to achieve somewhat more than I expected. For all those who now call themselves Erasistrateans have come round to the opposite opinion, and are lining up all and sundry to be phlebotomised.'[53] Now it is made quite clear in *On His Own Books* that this dissemination of the first work took place only after his first sojourn in Rome was over. 'Then, I can't say how, when I came to Rome the second time, summoned by the emperors, the man who had taken the book had died, and many people had got posses-sion of it.'[54] This shows that throughout Galen's first stay in Rome (162–6) Teuthras was alive, and kept the book, as best he could, as a confidential document; when Galen returned in 169, however, he was dead, and the book was common property. Teuthras, then, died

[52] For an estimate of Galen's speed of literary composition, see Smith (1979), p. 97n.
[53] K xi, 194–5. [54] K xix, 14–15.

between 166 and 169,[55] and the dissemination of the first work took place at once, since when Galen returned to Rome a number of people already had it. By the time the second work was written all the neo-Erasistrateans were hard at it, venesecting everyone in sight; and this was a direct result of the first work becoming available. Some years must have passed, no doubt, before a substantial proportion of the Erasistrateans were converted in this way, considering how radical was the change in their opinions; and it is further reasonable to suppose that Galen, a very busy man, did not find leisure to compose the second work, his Stesichorean recantation, until some time after the problem with the converted Erasistrateans had become acute. Hence, it would seem, the composition of the second work cannot be dated at the very beginning of Galen's second sojourn in Rome; some years at least must have elapsed before it was written, but it seems reasonable still to place it, as Ilberg does, in the time of Marcus Aurelius, up to 180. A relatively late date of composition is further supported by the fact, attested by the third work,[56] that under Severus the Erasistrateans still held their new opinions; Galen's recantation in his second work had evidently not had time to convert them back again to their old ones, or even to Galen's own now very moderate views on the place of venesection. Whether it ever did, of course, there is no way of knowing.

Galen refers in the second work to one unusual event, of which, unfortunately, there is probably no other record. This is the consumption of snow-water by Roman women.[57] If this was due to an unusually severe winter, and not merely a passing fad, it would help to date the work if the year could be identified. Apart from contemporary records, tree-rings can be used to identify severe winters; unfortunately, however, they provide no evidence for southern Europe for the period in question.[58]

One further clue is available. This is Diodorus the grammarian, who had a fit when his stomach was empty.[59] He was a man of some importance, since affairs of state required his attendance in the assembly. On Galen's diet he remained many years (ἐτῶν πολλῶν) in good health. If we allow a year or two after Galen's first arrival in Rome for him to get a patient of distinction (say 165; by 169 he was hobnobbing with emperors) we can date the second work, at the

---

[55] This information might be useful for dating Galen's *Glossary* (for the problem, see Smith (1979) p. 160).
[56] K xi, 253.   [57] K xi, 205.
[58] I am grateful to Mr D. J. Underhill, University of East Anglia, for information on tree-ring dating.
[59] K xi, 242.

earliest, 'many years' after 165. The only question is what 'many years' means. To suppose ten gives a date of 175 at the earliest for the second work, which agrees well with that suggested by the earlier argument.

The most notable development and change in Galen's views and methods, then, took place between the composition of the first and second works on venesection, a period probably of ten or fifteen years. The third work on venesection is not very informative on development, except, as already mentioned, in showing that right to the end of his life he maintained his somewhat individualistic opinions on sites for revulsive venesection. The work is otherwise very valuable in providing an extensive summary of all Galen's mature opinions on venesection, with an appendix on arteriotomy for good measure. The medical reader of it cannot but be impressed with Galen's skill and thoroughness as a clinician. In it, Galen is scarcely polemical at all, and it would be pleasing to think that he grew in charity towards his colleagues with advancing age, as the works on venesection seem to show. It is outside the scope of this study, however, to discuss this somewhat doubtful proposition.

CHAPTER 6

Galen, venesection and the Hippocratic Corpus

At the beginning of his first work on venesection Galen expresses his surprise that Erasistratus, a man so punctilious in matters of detail, should have mentioned venesection only once in all his works, and at that only in passing; for, says Galen, it is a remedy of such strength and efficacy that it was regarded by the ancients as nothing less than the most effective of all.[1] It is made clear later[2] that the ancients to whom he refers are, in fact, Erasistratus' predecessors in the profession, including Hippocrates; Galen frequently mentions Hippocrates' use of the remedy in this work, observing that he employed it in most diseases and in the most acute,[3] and that even Asclepiades, who rejected almost all the other methods of Hippocrates, nevertheless still made use of venesection.[4] In another work Galen maintains that venesection has been dealt with very completely by Hippocrates.[5] He is not alone in this opinion. Littré observes: 'When we enquire which remedies, among the many that were used, are most frequently mentioned as having been applied, we find that bloodletting and the evacuants – emetics and, in particular, purgatives – play the principal role in the therapy of the Hippocratic physicians, and hence of Hippocrates himself.'[6] Adams expresses a similar opinion in his commentary on Paulus Aegineta. 'We have had occasion frequently to remark', he says, 'that Hippocrates practised venesection freely in various diseases. He has left no treatise, however, expressly on the subject.'[7]

The impression conveyed by both these nineteenth-century writers, and by Galen himself, is that the Hippocratic writers frequently

---

[1] K xi, 147–8. See also Caelius Aurelianus, *CD.* ii.53: 'At the start of treatment (of paralysis) Erasistratus recommends an enema, neglecting the power of phlebotomy, although among the ancients no remedy was more highly esteemed.'
[2] K xi, 149.   [3] K xi, 150.   [4] K xi, 163.   [5] K xiv, 665.
[6] L 2, 390 (translated). This passage occurs in Littré's introduction to his text and translation of the *Appendix* to *Regimen in Acute Diseases*. As will be shown, this *Appendix* is the only work in the Corpus that gives any support at all to such an assertion.
[7] *The seven books of Paulus Aegineta*, tr. F. Adams (1847) vol. ii, p. 319. Francis Adams (1796–1861) was a Scottish country practitioner who also translated part of the Hippocratic corpus (*The genuine works of Hippocrates*, 1849).

mentioned venesection, and used it freely. If this is so, then Galen, in making liberal use of it, is merely carrying on an old and distinguished tradition. But is it so? There is no doubt that Galen would have wished his practices to have the approval of Hippocrates, whom he regarded as little short of a god; but Galen may not be above creating his gods in his own image. Did the Hippocratic writers, in fact, give great prominence to venesection? The question is important for any study of the origins and development of Galen's ideas on the subject.

The Hippocratic corpus, in Littré's edition, fills with its text and French translation the better part of nine large volumes. In the whole collection there are only about seventy references to bloodletting, all of them brief; there is scarcely one that occupies more than a few lines of the text, and many take up only one. They may be summarised as follows.

In those most Hippocratic of the seven books of the *Epidemics*, I and III,[8] there are no references to venesection in the former and only one in the latter;[9] a patient with fever was bled from the arm and his pain was relieved. Book II has rather more to offer. The maidservant of Stymargos, to whom Galen refers in the bloodletting works and elsewhere,[10] had no lochial discharge after childbirth; although she had tremor of the whole body she was bled from the ankle, and recovered.[11] The six other references to the remedy in this work are all brief. Venesection is recommended in flatulence,[12] in sphacelus,[13] in sudden loss of speech without fever,[14] in fracture of the skull,[15] and in hydrops with cough;[16] there is also a practical hint on the use of a tourniquet.[17] *Epidemics* IV has one brief mention of a patient with a testicular lesion and cough, cured by venesection.[18] *Epidemics* V refers to a patient with abdominal pain and rumbling who was bled from either arm alternately until exsanguinated (ἔξαιμος); he recovered.[19] The remedy was also used in two patients with disease of the hip,[20] from one of whom a large amount of blood was abstracted;[21] this patient and the one who was alleged to have been exsanguinated are the only ones mentioned in the Corpus as having blood removed in

---

[8] The opinion is Galen's (K VII, 890). The interesting question of which works in the Corpus Galen regarded as genuinely Hippocratic, if indeed it can be answered at all, is outside the scope of this work, though it will be mentioned incidentally. See J. Mewaldt, 'Galenos über echte und unechte Hippocratica', *Hermes* 44 (1905) 111–34; H. Diller, 'Zur Hippokratesauffassung des Galen', *Hermes* 68 (1933) 167–82; Bardong; and especially Smith, *The Hippocratic tradition*.

[9] L 3, 124.   [10] K VII, 602–4, and translation, K 161–2.   [11] L 5, 126.
[12] L 5, 130.   [13] L 5, 132.   [14] L 5, 130.   [15] L 5, 129.   [16] L 5, 130.
[17] L 5, 116.   [18] L 5, 196.   [19] L 5, 206.   [20] L 5, 206, 208.
[21] L 5, 206.

large quantities. There are a further five references to venesection in the fifth book, too inconspicuous to have been noticed by the compiler of Littré's index.[22] *Epidemics* VI has a patient bled from the sublingual veins without effect,[23] and it advises opening a vein in the popliteal region for urinary affections in young patients.[24] Book VII mentions that a patient with headache had some relief from the remedy.[25]

There are eight brief references to venesection in the *Aphorisms*. If used in pregnancy it causes abortion;[26] ruptures extending to the back from the elbows are relieved by venesection;[27] pain in the eyes is treated with venesection,[28] and the internal vein at the elbow is to be opened for dysuria.[29] One should bleed patients in the springtime.[30] Each of the last three aphorisms appears in two places in the work. The remedy is mentioned seven times in the *Coan Prenotions*. Three references are to conditions in which it is harmful.[31,32,33] A fourth says that chest pains that are not relieved by venesection go on to empyema.[34] Venesection relieves when there is abdominal pain and swelling without fever,[35] and it is beneficial when bleeding from haemorrhoids or from the nose has been imprudently suppressed, leading to paralysis or spasm.[36]

The anatomy of the veins – or rather the supposed anatomy[37] – is dealt with in *Nature of Man*[38] and in the tract with the inappropriate title *Nature of Bones*;[39] both these works briefly mention preferred sites for venesection. There is one brief reference to venesection in each of the treatises *On Wounds*,[40] *On Sevens*,[41] *Humours*,[42] *Prorrhetic*,[43] *Airs, Waters, Places*,[44] *Prognostic*,[45] *Physician*,[46] and *Diseases of Women*.[47] *Places in Man* has three references. A particular vein is recommended for bleeding in diseases of the spleen.[48] Bleeding from the limbs is recommended in angina,[49] and venesection is mentioned for head-

---

[22] L 5, 242, 244, 244, 250, 252.   [23] L 5, 336.   [24] L 5, 268.

[25] L 5, 447. The description resembles one of meningitis.

[26] L 4, 542.

[27] L 4, 568. Galen (K XVIIIa, 34) suggests that for 'ruptures' one should read 'pains', which makes better sense.

[28] L 4, 570, 590.

[29] L 4, 572. Galen (K XVIIIa, 57) thinks this aphorism is an interpolation, since it was Hippocratic practice to bleed only from the leg in genito-urinary diseases.

[30] L 4, 574, 592.   [31] L 5, 656.   [32] L 5, 658.   [33] L 5, 692.   [34] L 5, 668.

[35] L 5, 648.   [36] L 5, 656.

[37] Mewaldt refers to it, with justice, as a 'wunderliche Aderbeschreibung'.

[38] L 6, 58–60.   [39] L 9, 174–8.   [40] L 6, 430.   [41] L 8, 652.   [42] L 5, 502.

[43] L 5, 564.   [44] L 2, 78.   [45] L 2, 146–8.   [46] L 9, 214.   [47] L 8, 172.

[48] L 6, 282.

[49] L 6, 322. Angina in antiquity was an inflammatory condition of the neck and fauces.

ache.[50] In *Diseases* I it is used in empyema.[51] *Diseases* III has two references; for ileus, bleed from the head and elbow,[52] and in angina, take blood from the sublingual veins and also from the elbow if strength permits.[53] *Affections* recommends bleeding from the nostrils or frontal vein in diseases of the head,[54] and where the spleen is enlarged one should bleed from the vein called splenitis.[55] In *Internal Diseases* the physician is recommended to start treatment with bloodletting in certain diseases of the lung,[56] and in jaundice to bleed from the elbow; the side is not specified.[57] The side is prescribed, however, in disease of the spleen, where the internal vein at the left elbow should be used;[58] and in hepatitis, where the corresponding vein on the right is recommended if medicinal treatment fails.[59] The work *On Vision* approves of venesection for certain eye diseases[60] but not for others.[61]

The first part of *Regimen in Acute Diseases*[62] contains two references to venesection, both concerning pain in the chest. This must be relieved by bloodletting or purgation before ptisan is administered, or the patient will die;[63] and in treating it the inner vein of the forearm should be opened and blood allowed to flow until it becomes either redder or livid.[64]

The last work to be considered is the *Appendix* to *Regimen in Acute Diseases*. Littré regarded this appendix as spurious, and Jones, in the Loeb Hippocrates, although translating the main work, made no mention of the appendix at all. Galen, however, thought that parts of it were by Hippocrates, or worthy of him.[65] It appears to be a lengthy

---

[50] L 6, 330.   [51] L 6, 164.   [52] L 7, 134.   [53] L 7, 130.   [54] L 6, 210.
[55] L 6, 230.   [56] L 7, 178.   [57] L 7, 258.   [58] L 7, 250.   [59] L 7, 242.
[60] L 9, 160.   [61] L 9, 152.
[62] So called to distinguish it from the *Appendix*.   [63] L 2, 258–60.
[64] L 2, 272. Galen comments on this, with a long account of the anatomy of the veins, at K xv, 527ff. (*Commentary on Regimen in Acute Diseases*).
[65] Galen (K xv, 763), in his commentary on the passage from the *Appendix* cited below, n. 67, says it is worthy of Hippocrates, and expresses his surprise that it was not included in the *Aphorisms*. In the *De Methodo Medendi* (K x, 286–7), he attributes to Hippocrates the discovery of the indication for venesection from the severity of the disease, to which the passage above refers. The idea does not appear elsewhere in the Corpus, although Galen (K x, 288–9) says that Hippocrates expresses it in all his works and in his treatise on ulcers, in which he says that purgation (with cathartics) is called for in patients with a variety of traumatic and other conditions. Galen is less complimentary, however, about some of the other parts of the *Appendix*. In commenting on the passage on hydrops mentioned in n. 75 below he observes 'The man who wrote this is manifestly in error' (K xv, 891); and again, on the diet recommended (L 2, 498–500) for the phlebotomised patient, he says: 'His practice of giving warm loaves soaked in red wine and oil to the phlebotomised patient to eat is stupid and out-of-date' (K xv, 893). Galen has some comments on the genuineness of this work in general in his commentary (K xv, 732–4). Many doctors, he says, suspected that it is not by Hippocrates, though it had been suggested that it was the work of a disciple, or that it might represent notes towards a book not completed in Hippocrates'

collection of notes, mostly somewhat disjointed. It does, however, provide some evidence – perhaps the only evidence – for the contention of Galen, Adams and Littré that Hippocrates was an enthusiastic and copious bloodletter. The material in it will therefore be dealt with in rather more detail.

This *Appendix*, which occupies with the French translation 134 pages in Littré's edition, contains eight references to venesection, one of which may be the source of Galen's idea that the men of old regarded it as the most important of all remedies. The passage, after listing a number of conditions, continues: καὶ ξυστροφαὶ νουσημάτων, οὐ δύνανται λύεσθαι, ἤν τις πρῶτον ἐπιχειρέῃ φαρμακεύειν· ἀλλὰ φλεβοτομίη τῶν τοιῶνδε ἡγεμονικόν ἐστιν· ἔπειτα δὲ ἐπὶ κλυσμάν, ἢν μὴ μέγα καὶ ἰσχυρὸν τὸ νούσημα ᾖ· εἰ δὲ μή, καὶ ὕστερον φαρμακείης δεῖ. δέεται δὲ ἀσφαλείης καὶ μετριότητος μετὰ φαρμακείης φλεβοτομίη.[66] Which Littré translates: 'Enfin les maladies aiguës où il y a des engorgements d'humeurs, ne se résolvent pas si on les attaque d'abord par la purgation. La saignée en est le remède capital; ensuite on en vient aux clystères, à moins que l'affection ne soit grande et intense; si elle l'est, une purgation est nécessaire après la saignée; mais la saignée avec la purgation a besoin de précautions et de modération.' (In fact, acute diseases, where there is engorgement with humours, are not resolved if the first treatment is with purgatives. For these, bloodletting is the principal remedy; thereafter one has recourse to enemas, at least where the disease is slight and not severe; where it is severe, a purgative is necessary after the bleeding.

lifetime, to which others had subsequently added. Some of the sentiments in it are entirely worthy of Hippocrates and resemble his own expression and his thought; others resemble his work in one of these respects but not the other, and others again are like him in neither of these respects. It is sometimes hard to avoid the conclusion that Galen was in the habit of attributing to Hippocrates any passage in the Corpus with which he happened at the time to agree; this thesis has been convincingly argued by Smith in his work *The Hippocratic tradition.* Galen regards the work *Nature of Man,* for example, as a very fine work by Hippocrates himself (K II, 132), but the description of the veins in it is not, he says elsewhere, by Hippocrates (K V, 529). He quotes the opening sentence of *Nutriment* as a genuine utterance (K II, 26); yet *Aphorisms* (see above) is also genuine, except for some interpolations. It apparently does not occur to Galen that these two works are strange bedfellows in style and content.

[66] L 2, 400–2. There is some doubt about the Greek text, with a number of possible MS readings. Both Littré and the modern edition of R. Joly, *Hippocrate* vol. VI pt. 2 (1972) 69–70, appeal to Galen's commentary (K XV, 774) in which he makes the point that the meaning of the whole passage is that phlebotomy should be used first, and purgation, if at all, only after phlebotomy has been performed. Joly, following the Greek as Galen quotes it (K XV, 769) therefore reads μετὰ φλεβοτομίην φαρμακείη, 'purgation after phlebotomy', whereas Littré favours μετὰ φαρμακείης φλεβοτομίη 'phlebotomy in combination with purgation'. The sense of the passage is much the same with either reading.

But one must use bloodletting in combination with purgation with caution and in moderation.)

Another passage relevant to Galen's practice occurs earlier in the same section: 'In the acute diseases you will phlebotomise if the disease appears severe, and the patients are in the prime of life and in possession of strength.'[67] It goes on to say that in pleuritis, if the patient is debilitated and much blood has already been taken, an enema should be administered. Further indications are found in the following passage, which refers to pneumonia and pleuritis: 'If the pain should extend upwards towards the clavicle or round the breast, or to the region of the arm, it is necessary to cut the internal vein in the arm on whichever side is affected. Remove a quantity according to the bodily habitus and the season and time of life and colour, boldly going as far as loss of consciousness if the pain is severe. Next give an enema.'[68] This introduces several factors that must be considered when deciding on the measure of the evacuation: physical type, time of year, patient's age, and his complexion. Galen remarks that both the colour of the patient's complexion and of the issuing blood provide information.[69] The venesection must take place on the affected side of the body;[70] there are three other references in the Corpus to this requirement,[71] to which Galen attached much importance.[72] And the removal of blood, when the pain is severe, must be continued until the patient loses consciousness; this is the only reference in the Corpus to such a practice, if we exclude the patient already mentioned who was allegedly rendered bloodless.[73] Galen makes much of all these indications.[74]

A further passage refers to hydropic patients. Where there is anasarca the physician can do nothing; when, however, the hydrops is combined with emphysema, then, if the patient is breathless, and it is summer, and he is in the prime of life and strong, one may take blood from the arm.[75] Similarly, when there is loss of speech in acute diseases, one should bleed from the internal vein of the right arm, the quantity taken depending on the constitution and age of the patient.[76] There is a reference to venesection from the arm and sublingual veins in angina with imminent suffocation,[77] and one to venesection in the spasms of tetanus.[78] Lastly, some precautions to be observed by

---

[67] L 2, 398. [68] L 2, 458–60. [69] K xi, 172.
[70] The Greek, however, is not altogether clear.
[71] See nn. 55, 58, 59 above. [72] See, e.g., K xi, 284, 295ff.
[73] L 5, 206. I take ἔξαιμος to mean that the flow of blood ceased, not that he had none left, or the outcome would have been less happy.
[74] E.g. K xi, 267. [75] L 2, 498. [76] L 2, 404, 406. [77] L 2, 412.
[78] L 2, 468–70.

bloodletters are mentioned; before blood is taken the patient's bowels should be constipated, and he should abstain from wine.[79]

It may now be asked whether these references in the Corpus support the opinion that venesection was the major weapon in the Hippocratic armamentarium, or that, as Galen says, it was regarded by the ancients as the most effective of all remedies. It is mentioned only about seventy times in the entire Corpus. This, however, might mean only that the Hippocratic writers seldom mentioned any therapy at all, and this, as will be shown, is true of some of the works. But is venesection mentioned more frequently than that other standby of the Hippocratic physician, the purgative, or such other remedies as he had at his disposal? We may consider first the work that gives most attention to venesection, the *Appendix* to *Regimen in Acute Diseases*. This contains eight references to it. Purgatives and therapeutic purgations, however, are mentioned twenty times; enemas eleven; fomentations and plasters ten; expectorants four, and vomits, gargles and unctions four times. In the *Aphorisms* the pattern is the same; venesection is mentioned eight times, drugs purging upwards and downwards 32 times. The supposedly genuine part of *Regimen in Acute Diseases* concerns chiefly articles of diet, such as ptisan, oxymel and hydromel. None the less, to set against its two references to venesection it has three to purgatives, two to fomentations, and one to a suppository. In the *Coan Prenotions* there are seven references to venesection, but ten to purgatives. *Epidemics* v, with its eight references to venesection, has 32 to purgatives alone. The total, in these works, of 33 references to venesection must be set against 97 – nearly three times as many – to purgatives alone, without taking into account any of the other remedies mentioned in them. The work entitled *Diseases of Women* shows the same pattern in ancient gynaecology, but here the predominance of remedies other than bloodletting is particularly noticeable. It makes one mention of venesection, which it recommends in prolonged labour; this covers five or six lines of the text. There are, however, almost innumerable references to other remedies in this work, including purgatives, pessaries, fumigations, drinks, phlegmagogues, cholagogues, astringents, plasters and preparations for general medical use; it would be quite impracticable to list them. The author of this work, it is clear, did not regard venesection as the most effective of all remedies; nor could one possibly maintain, as one might of the author of *Epidemics* i and iii, that he did too little for his patients.

It would appear, then, that there is no evidence that the Hippocratic

[79] L 2, 508.

writers gave the principal place to venesection in any of their works. Only in the *Appendix* to *Regimen in Acute Diseases* is it accorded some prominence as a means of treatment, and even here it receives only eight brief mentions in the 67 pages of Greek text. No work in the Corpus is chiefly, or even in any appreciable part, devoted to the subject, and this in spite of the fact that it was one of the very few therapeutic agents that the general physician of Hippocratic times had at his disposal. It cannot be denied that the Hippocratic physicians, or most of them, used the remedy; that they regarded it as the most effective of all, however, and that Hippocrates dealt at length with it, is simply not true.[80] Either Galen is referring to other ancient authorities, whose works are now lost, when he maintains that the old physicians did so regard it, or he is attributing to Hippocrates opinions that the authors of the Corpus never held.

This opinion is in conflict, not only with that of Galen and Adams, but with that of so great a Hippocratic scholar as Littré. His view would seem clear enough from his translation of the passage, already quoted, from the *Appendix*.[81] He renders ἀλλὰ φλεβοτομίη τῶν τοιῶνδε ἡγεμονικόν ἐστιν by 'la saignée en est le remède capital', a word that can only mean the chief or most important remedy. In his introduction to the text, however, he makes a curious mistake, giving the impression that he is quoting his translation from memory. 'Le traitement capital', he says, 'et, comme dit l'auteur, celui qui doit précéder tous les autres, ἡγεμονικόν, est la saignée.'[82] From his use of the conjunction *et* it appears that he thought the author had said, not only that venesection was the capital remedy, but also that it was ἡγεμονικόν, a word which Littré here (correctly, I think) renders by 'celui qui doit précéder tous les autres'; it might be most literally rendered in English by 'leading'. But the Hippocratic author does not say this. He uses only one adjective, ἡγεμονικόν, and I think it is clear from the context that it means the leading remedy only in that sense that it is the one that must come first in time. He makes it clear that purgatives must not be used *first*; the first remedy to be used is phlebotomy, and thereafter enemas or purges. As has already been shown, this was Galen's interpretation of the passage also. Littré and Adams both wrote at a time when venesection was, in fact, the chief remedy used by many physicians in the acute fevers;[83] but the sacred canon, rightly interpreted, gives no support to this heresy.

[80] I was unaware until Smith's book appeared that Le Clerc, in his 1729 history of medicine, had made the same point (Smith (1979) pp. 21–2).

[81] L 2, 400–2.   [82] L 2, 380

[83] See, for example, R. J. Graves, *Clinical lectures on the practice of medicine* (1884) vol. i, p. 357; his first edition dates from 1843.

This view of the place of venesection in the Corpus is not original. It was put forward in the seventeenth century by Bauda, although his argument was different. He says:

Anyone who cares to go through the works of Hippocrates will observe a considerable number of diseases, and of patients, mentioned, which he has treated without letting blood. For example when he speaks of pleurisy, and the means of treating it, he makes hardly any mention of this remedy, which is held, at the present time, not only to be the most certain mode of treatment, but indeed the only one. On the rare occasions when he does employ it, it is with great caution and restraint, and he is very far from making it his principal remedy.[84]

This could not be better put, but now Bauda weakens his case by appealing to *Epidemics* i and iii, the very works that provide the least support for it. He says: 'In his book of epidemic diseases he reports 42 patients, attacked by diseases so violent and so dangerous that of this number only 17 survived; in this whole book, however, he mentions only one patient who was bled.'[85] It is clear that i and iii, the books among the *Epidemics* most universally accepted as genuine, are the ones referred to; the total of 42 patients makes this certain. Now it is perfectly true that there is only one mention of venesection among the 42 cases; the extraordinary thing about these works, however, is that hardly any other means of treatment is ever mentioned either.[86] In *Epidemics* i we find brief mention of one enema, two suppositories, one purge, and two pessaries; in book iii, two purges and one suppository. These works present a mystery that cannot be considered here. For most of the patients no treatment whatever is mentioned. It might be argued that the author did nothing except to observe the patients. But if so, his aim must have been to note and describe scientifically the course of their illnesses, and this must have been affected by treatment. It is unthinkable that someone was not providing it; hence it should have been mentioned. If it was given, but the author did not think it worth mentioning because he believed it to be without effect, he had no business to be a doctor. Bauda is carried away by his argument here and says: 'One cannot but consider what Hippocrates reports concerning the remedies he had administered to these patients. There he makes mention of washing, fomentations, baths and similar remedies, without leaving anything out; yet he does not speak of bloodletting at all, except for one patient.'[87] This is not so; the

[84] A. Bauda, *Discours curieux contre l'abus des saigneés* (c.1672), pp. 10ff. (translated).
[85] Bauda, loc. cit.
[86] It was no doubt these works that caused Asclepiades to describe Hippocratic medicine as an exercise in death (K xi, 163).
[87] Bauda, pp. 14–15.

fact is that practically nothing in the way of treatment, whether by venesection or any other means, is mentioned at all in these two works. Bauda's general thesis, however, is correct. Like Galen, he is an interested party; and he has not hesitated to select from the works of the prince of physicians material to support his view.

This illustrious physician [he says of Galen], writing to his friend Glaucus, and instructing him in his method for the treatment of fevers, says nothing at all to him about the necessity of letting blood, except for quartan fever; and here, moreover, he advises him to use it with great circumspection. His books on therapeutic method[88] are full of accounts of patients in whom bloodletting would seem to have been necessary, but where he has omitted to administer this remedy.[89]

As has been shown, Galen's views on venesection changed somewhat in the course of time, and it is possible to support almost any thesis by making judicious selections from his works. Bauda, however, needed the still enormous authority of Galen to counter the alarming excesses of bloodletting which, if we can believe him, were taking place in France in his time.[90]

It is clear, then, that Galen – at the time of his first work on venesection at least – was an enthusiastic venesectionist, and appealed to the ancients for support for his opinions. The Hippocratic corpus, at least, provides no support for his contention that vene-section was regarded by the ancients as the most effective of all remedies; Bauda was perfectly right in maintaining that the Hippo-cratic writers used it only occasionally, and with moderation. Where, then, did Galen's opinions come from? Were they to some extent peculiar to him, or were they typical of educated medical opinion some centuries after Hippocrates? Before an attempt can be made to answer this question it will be necessary to summarise Galen's views on venesection.

---

[88] *De Methodo Medendi* (K x, 1–1021).   [89] Bauda, p. 15.
[90] Bauda (p. 55) observes: 'Nevertheless, against the advice of Galen and the whole drift of his arguments, more blood is shed by venesection in one town of this realm, in a single day, than is let in a whole year in all the provinces of Germany put together.'

CHAPTER 7

Galen's practice of venesection

It has been shown in the previous chapter that although the Hippo-cratic writers unquestionably made use of venesection, they mention it only briefly and in passing, neither offering a rational explanation for its use nor listing the indications. Galen is more systematic. From a study of all his references to venesection it is possible to extract a good deal of information on his practice, and to determine not only what he did but also sometimes why he did it.[1] His indications will be considered first.

In brief, Galen regards venesection as an evacuant remedy to be used in certain patients with plethos, though not in all. Suppression of wonted evacuations of blood, such as the menses or bleeding piles, may lead to plethos, which in turn, if not dispersed, may result in inflammation. Apart from these considerations, any severe disease is an indication for venesection, not only when established, but even when foreseen or expected; thus venesection may be used prophylac-tically in healthy subjects. Galen employs the remedy widely in fever. It is further used as a revulsive or derivative remedy, to direct blood away from or towards a particular part; and a number of pathological conditions are specifically mentioned in which it is applied. These indications will now be considered in more detail.

As an evacuant, Galen says, venesection is selective; it empties only the veins, whereas starvation leads to the evacuation of the whole body, a process attended with many troubles for the patient. Besides, venesection acts at once, whereas starvation is slow[2] and the weakest

---

[1] There is some account of Galen's practice of venesection in J. Bauer, *Geschichte der Aderlässe* (1870), pp. 68ff., which is disappointingly rhetorical and says more about Galen's pathology than his use of the remedy. A better, though brief, account is in the introduction to *Andreas Vesalius Bruxellensis: the bloodletting letter of 1539*, ed. J. B. de C. M. Saunders and C. D. O'Malley (n.d.) pp. 10–15. P. H. Niebyl, 'Galen, van Helmont, and blood letting', and R. E. Siegel, 'Galen's concept of bloodletting in relation to his ideas on pulmonary and peripheral blood flow and blood formation', in *Science, medicine and society in the Renaissance*, ed. A. G. Debus (1972), provide some incidental references to Galen's methods, marred in Siegel's paper by his desire to show that Galen knew the pulmonary circulation.

[2] K xi, 156–7.

of all evacuant remedies;[3] Galen remarks later that it does not evacuate directly at all.[4] In many patients, then, who have an established plethos of blood, Galen recommends venesection; the Erasistrateans, who at the time of Galen's first arrival in Rome totally abjured it, made use only of starvation and bandaging of the limbs.[5] Venesection, in Galen's view, is a lifesaving procedure in some plethoric patients; he mentions specifically two patients treated by Erasistratus without it, who, he says, would not have died had it been employed.[6] In a later work, however, he admits that starvation and other remedies may be called for, rather than venesection, in some plethoric patients.[7]

Venesection as an evacuant can remove two kinds of bad blood: blood that is intrinsically bad, in that it does not perform the primary function of blood, which is to nourish, and blood that is bad by virtue of being in excess in a particular part of the body, constituting a plethos.[8] It may be dangerous, however, to try to remove intrinsically bad blood by venesection. In patients suffering from lassitude, says Galen, there is not much good blood, but an abundance of crude or unconcocted humours; if peripheral blood is taken away by venesection, it will only be replaced by worse blood spreading outwards from the first veins to take its place.[9] Galen's ideas of plethos have already been discussed (p. 12). He recognises two kinds: dynamic plethos, which is due to weakness of the natural eliminative faculty or dynamis, and a more mechanical variety, plethos by filling, in which the vessels are physically distended by the excess of blood being poured into them. Some physicians, he says, deny this variety, believing all plethos to be dynamic;[10] others recognise only the mechanical variety. Chief among these latter are the materialists such as Asclepiades, who reject the natural faculties.[11] Erasistratus also accepted only this variety, plethos by filling, and called it plethora, a term restricted also by Galen to this variety.[12] Galen explains how residues move from part to part until they find one that is too feeble in its excretory faculty to reject them; there they establish themselves. Thus the parts with the weakest excretory powers are the most liable to accumulate residues.[13] A plethos is thus set up, and both varieties

---

[3] K xi, 178.[4] K xi, 185.[5] K xi, 187ff.[6] K xi, 205–6.

[7] K x, 287ff. Chapter 5 deals with the changes, in the course of time, in Galen's attitude to the Erasistrateans.

[8] K x, 640.[9] K vi, 263.[10] K vii, 520–1.[11] K vii, 515.

[12] K vii, 538–9. I therefore use the term plethos when referring to the phenomenon in general.

[13] K xi, 274–5. The ancient idea of movement of residues persists; a soldier once told me that he was suffering from a rush of shit to the brain, a condition mentioned by Galen (K vi, 295).

of plethos require evacuation[14] if further mischief is to be prevented: putrefaction of the compacted humour in dynamic plethos, rupture of blood vessels in the variety due to filling.[15] When the plethos consists of overheated blood, there is further danger of fever; it should therefore be evacuated without delay, since further complications may be introduced if the plethos changes its seat and invades some vital organ of the body.[16] Not all concourses of humours, however, necessarily require either venesection or purgation; starvation, baths, exercises and rubbings may be the appropriate treatment for some.[17] And, as we shall see, venesection is often necessary in the absence of a plethoric concourse of humours; to make plethos the only indication, as Menodotus did, is wrong.[18] When venesection is to be employed in plethos, however, there is no need to wait until complications set in; it may be used early, when the only abnormality is a local redundancy of humour.[19]

Although Galen develops the doctrine of perittomatic diseases, he did not originate it;[20] it is frequently implied in the Hippocratic corpus and by other ancient writers. Certain natural, or supposedly natural, evacuations are regarded as highly beneficial by writers in antiquity, and it is a source of concern to the physician if they do not appear when they ought to.[21] Hence Galen's alarm when the Erasistrateans refused to venesect the woman mentioned at the beginning of his second work on venesection, whose menses had not appeared for

---

[14] K xi, 259.   [15] K xi, 266.   [16] K xi, 287.   [17] K x, 287ff.
[18] K xv, 766; K xviiia, 575–6.   [19] K x, 778–9.
[20] R. O. Steuer and J. B. de C. M. Saunders, *Ancient Egyptian and Cnidian medicine* (1959), have speculatively suggested that the idea of disease originating from residues and their putrefaction is of Egyptian origin.
[21] Examples from the Hippocratic corpus: A woman vomiting blood was cured by the menses breaking out (L 4, 542). Haemorrhoids protect against a number of diseases (L 5, 304). A certain Alcippus was warned not to have his piles treated, but did so; he went mad (L 5, 196). The surgeon is warned at least twice in the Corpus to leave one pile untreated when ligating haemorrhoids (L 2, 516; L 4, 566). Suppression of the menses leads to epilepsy and other diseases (L 5, 702), and their appearance results in the cure of peripneumonia (L 5, 452). In barren women, vomiting of blood promotes conception (L 5, 708). Pains in the head and neck are cured by haemor-rhages (L 5, 566). Fevers are dissipated by epistaxis occurring on certain days (L 5, 614), and if nose-bleeding is stopped the patient suffers spasms, which are relieved by bloodletting (L 5, 564).
    Aretaeus says that in cholera the suppression of the diarrhoea is undesirable, since undigested matters are being desirably eliminated (vi.4.1). (The treatment of diarrhoea with castor oil persisted into the twentieth century.) Cachexia, he says, may result from suppression of bleeding from haemorrhoids (iii.16.3). Haemorrhage from the nose is favourable in peripneumonia (ii.1.4). Some patients periodically pass bloody urine, and if this discharge is suppressed they suffer from various diseases (iv.3.8).
    Celsus mentions that arthritis of the hands and feet is rare in women unless the menses have been suppressed (iv.31.1).

several months; sure enough, she became more and more dyspnoeic until she suffocated.[22] Galen explains that the lung is one of the organs that is feebly endowed with the excretory faculty, and hence is often unable to eject a plethos that settles in it.[23] But venesection, by removing the plethos, effects a cure. Galen says that this is shown by recent events in Rome, when many women drank snow-water and their menses were suppressed; but the doctors kept them in good health by venesecting them.[24] In suppression of the menses bloodletting should be the first remedy of all.[25] It is not always necessary, however, to open a vein; the menses may be brought on by scarifying the ankles.[26]

One of the dangers of plethos is inflammation. Galen deals at some length with Erasistratus' theory of inflammation, which he does not accept, in his first work on venesection. Erasistratus, unlike Galen, believed that the arteries in health contained pneuma but no blood. Both the arteries and the veins divided into smaller and smaller branches, finally ending in minute passages having orifices that were normally closed to liquids. If, however, there was a plethos of blood in the veins, their ends might be forced open and the blood might pass across to the arteries, leading to fever and inflammation by obstructing the free passage of pneuma sent along by the heart. Inflammation was believed to follow trauma because the pneuma escaped from the injured arteries, leading to a transfer of blood from the veins to fill the empty space left in the arteries. The plethos, and the subsequent inflammation, were to be dispersed by emptying the veins; here Erasistratus and Galen are in agreement. They disagree, however, on the method to be used, for Erasistratus never employed venesection.[27] Galen also agreed with Erasistratus on the existence of the arterio-venous inosculations. But, says Galen, if Erasistratus is right, then nature has constructed these anastomoses for no other purpose than to promote inflammatory diseases; for such diseases could not exist, on the Erasistratean hypothesis, if there were no anastomoses.[28] Erasistratus proposed to empty the veins by starving the patient;

---

[22] K XI, 190.   [23] K XI, 275.

[24] K XI, 205. The deleterious qualities of ice-water are mentioned in the Hippocratic work *Airs, Waters, Places* (L 2, 36); they are doubtless imaginary, as the health of Americans bears witness. Winters in Rome severe enough to freeze the fountains are uncommon in modern times, but we know from Horace (*Odes* 1.9) that when Soracte was covered with snow the streams were frozen on his Sabine farm, admittedly at a higher altitude; he wisely preferred the local wine, however, to ice-water. On the other hand the practice of the Roman women may have been a fad rather than a result of necessity.

[25] K XI, 201.   [26] K XI, 283.   [27] K XI, 153ff.

[28] K III, 493–4. The work is the *De Usu Partium*, which is full of Galen's teleological concept of a nature that does nothing in vain. She made the arteriovenous inoscu-

Galen, in his first work on bloodletting at least, believed that the quickest and most effective way to empty them was by venesection.[29] The aim, once again, is to prevent inflammation; Galen's ideas on the pathogenesis, however, are somewhat different from those of Erasistratus. He is a perittomatist; in the *De Usu Partium* he says that the evacuation of the residues of nutriment is of crucial importance. If the residues accumulate they become hotter and more acrid, and so give rise to inflammations, erysipelas, herpes, carbuncles, fevers and numerous other conditions. To prevent this from happening, particularly in the important parts, nature has provided for the elimination of residues.[30] But where she is unable to achieve this alone, the physician must assist her; this is both a Hippocratic and a Galenic precept.[31] The treatment for a plethos of humours, Galen says, is evacuation; for evacuation is the opposite of plethos.[32] Inflammation (φλεγμονή) is due to an excess of blood of moderate viscosity in the affected part; this blood, initially at least, may be otherwise good.[33] But the blood that collects in the part does not remain good; it quickly becomes hot and bilious, putrefies, and the heat thus generated gives rise to fevers of various kinds.[34] Although trauma is one cause of inflammation of this sort, it can also arise spontaneously because of the weakness of the part or the strength of the residues; in a body abounding in residues the risk of inflammation is far greater than in one that has very little excess of nutriment.[35] Thick and glutinous foods, too, are more likely to promote inflammation; for the humours they generate, being more viscid, are more liable to impaction in the plethoric parts.[36] The flowing in of hot blood, which constitutes inflammation, ought to be repulsed at the beginning, thus discouraging it from later moving to some vital part where it may do great harm.[37]

The ill effects of inflammation are so great that the physician is

---

lations, he says, in order to confer the benefits of respiration and the pulse on the veins as well as the heart and arteries.

[29] K xi, 156. Later, as the second and third bloodletting works show, unexpected events caused him to modify somewhat the views of his youth.

[30] K iii, 686.　　[31] K xi, 170.

[32] K i, 99. The doctrine of the treatment of diseases with their opposites is, again, both Hippocratic and Galenic (K xi, 167). It was not, however, universally accepted in antiquity; the Hippocratic work *Epidemics* vi refers to one Herodicus who killed feverish patients with exercise and vapour baths (L 5, 302), and Celsus (iii.9.3) mentions Petron, who treated febrile patients by making them as hot as possible; many of them died.

[33] K xi, 73.　　[34] K ix, 693.

[35] K vii, 290–3; 387. The ancients' morbid fear of residues persists to this day, as is shown by the widespread use of laxatives to prevent dangers that do not in fact exist.

[36] K vii, 287–8.　　[37] K xii, 896.

justified, not only in letting blood when it is established, but in using venesection prophylactically before the plethos develops, for instance immediately after an injury.[38] Even the empiricists use it in this way when some part of the body has been bruised.[39] Trauma, however, is not the only indication. Galen recommends that certain patients, while still in good health, should be bled prophylactically at the approach of spring, provided that they are of temperate habits.[40] Venesection may also be used prophylactically on the suspicion that a severe disease may be impending.[41]

Galen uses phlebotomy extensively in fever, for which – or at least for the continuous variety – he has two main remedies, venesection and cooling drinks.[42] He believes, as mentioned in Chapter 1, in two principal mechanisms for fever. The first is an increased production of heat; the second is a failure of transpiration, preventing the heat from being dissipated. The body is innately hot; this heat is not generated by friction, as the atomists believe, and in fact it is the cause, not the result, of the movement of the arteries.[43] It is likewise the cause of growth.[44] Erasistratus, however, believed that no heat was innate, all being acquired from outside the body.[45] The arteries, according to Galen, pulsate in order to distribute the innate heat to every part of the body,[46] thus enabling the parts to grow; hence Galen's analogy of the hearth-fire, or perhaps more probably the hypocaust, which provided central heating to the Roman house.[47] As already shown, the production of good blood depends on the proper amount of heat being available for its formation. Such blood, however, may not remain good; if it becomes impacted in a plethoric part it may rot with the evolution of heat, which is one of the signs of inflammation.[48] Erasistratus went so far as to maintain that there was no fever without inflammation.[49] Galen says that heat thus generated in a part of the body may spread to the heart, which is the central furnace of the body, and make it hotter; when this happens the whole body becomes

---

[38] K x, 287ff.; K xv, 766; K xviiia, 575–6.

[39] For the same practice sixteen centuries later, see, for example, C. Waterton, *Essays on natural history* (1871): 'I consider inflammation to be the root and origin of all diseases. To subdue this at its earliest stage has been my constant care. Since my four-and-twentieth year I have been blooded above one hundred and ten times, in eighty of which I have performed the operation with my own hand' (pp. 42–3). When thrown from a mule in Demerara, he performed the operation as soon as consciousness returned: 'So I sat me down . . . took out my lancet, and drew some twenty ounces of blood from my arm. This prevented bad consequences, and put all to rights' (p. 199).

[40] K xi, 271–2; 281; 306. We learn from the Hippocratic work *Nature of Man* that blood increases in the spring.

[41] K xi, 277. [42] K x, 624–7. [43] K v, 703. [44] K xv, 155–6. [45] K xv, 14.

[46] K vii, 14–15. [47] K xi, 262; see above, p. 72. [48] K xi, 264.

[49] K xi, 226; Celsus iii.10.

feverish.[50] Fevers may, however, arise without any putrefaction of humours; this happens when the peccant humour cannot be transpired because the passages are obstructed. Galen believed that he could detect the signs of putrefaction in both the pulse and the urine, and that fever could occur in the absence of such signs, purely because of obstruction. But the obstructed humour, of course, is far more likely to putrefy as a result of its impaction, so that both mechanisms may operate together. The height of the fever, he says, is a measure of the severity of the obstruction.[51]

Since heat, which is in excess in fever, is augmented by food and drink, there is some theoretical justification for starving patients with fever, as long as fever is regarded, as it sometimes was in antiquity, as a disease in its own right. This was the Erasistratean treatment;[52] Galen implies that it sometimes killed the patient.[53] He sensibly remarks that one has to choose between feeding the patient and augmenting the fever, and starving him and reducing his strength. Unlike Erasistratus, however, he has the further remedy of venesection, which he uses to remove as much of the humour concerned as exceeds the normal level.[54] Having used venesection, he does not starve the patient as well;[55] no one, he says, would use both venesection and starvation.[56]

Galen hardly ever mentions the treatment of fevers by venesection without saying that certain conditions must be met before the treatment is employed. These will be dealt with at the end of this chapter. Bloodletting, he says, can be used in fevers due to obstruction, even where no signs of plethos exist,[57] as well as those caused by putrefaction of humours.[58] Venesection can extinguish the flame of continuous fevers,[59] in which it is particularly useful if the veins are distended.[60] It cools the body and abolishes or reduces the fever, particularly if pressed to the point of loss of consciousness. In the most powerful inflammations such copious evacuations, either by venesection or purgation, are the most effective remedies available.[61] In quartan fevers, where the blood, as commonly observed in diseases of the spleen, is thick and black, a vein in the left arm should be opened and blood removed until it becomes thin and yellowish.[62] Venesection

---

[50] K XI, 264–5. [51] K x, 564ff.

[52] K XI, 176–7; 190; 220. But Erasistratus believed that fever was a symptom rather than a disease in its own right (K XIV, 729).

[53] K XI, 182. [54] K x, 779. [55] K XI, 203–4.

[56] K XI, 247. The question whether Galen rather than Graves should have priority with the epitaph 'He Fed Fevers' is outside the scope of this work. For the practice of other authorities see, e.g., L 2, 302ff.; Celsus III.4.1–8, 16–17; Caelius, *AD* II.132–5.

[57] K x, 564–7. [58] K x, 777, 785. [59] K x, 637. [60] K XI, 41.

[61] K XVIIb, 445–6. [62] K XI, 38

should be undertaken when the paroxysms of fever are declining;[63] and when digestion is disturbed it should be postponed.[64]

Galen's principal indication for venesection, however, is a simple and all-embracing one: the severity of the patient's disease.[65] It has been mentioned already that he attributes the discovery of this indication to Hippocrates himself,[66] and he observes that venesection is used in most diseases and in the most acute.[67] He is careful to add, however, that the strength of the patient's faculties must be taken into account, together with other considerations; these will be dealt with subsequently. In various places Galen mentions specific conditions in which he uses venesection. These include angina and peripneumonia with suffocation,[68] synanche, suppression of the menses and of the haemorrhoidal flux,[69] and ophthalmia.[70] Galen refers to a patient with anorexia nervosa, successfully treated with venesection,[71] and he also uses the remedy in patients with dementia from vitiated humours, in hypermotility from heat, and – somewhat surprisingly – in torpor from cold.[72] He also employs it in the conventional manner, to cool a hot diathesis,[73] and he mentions in passing the following further conditions for which it is useful: gout, arthritis, epilepsy, melancholia, haemoptysis, scotomatic diseases, pleurisy and hepatitis.[74]

Finally, Galen makes use of bloodletting in order to divert blood from a particular part of the body. The two methods are known as παροχέτευσις, derivation, and ἀντίσπασις, revulsion. He describes the difference between them in the *De Methodo Medendi*. If bleeding from the mouth is brought to an end by a haemorrhage from the nose, this is derivation, since the flow is diverted to a nearby part; but if the haemorrhage that stops it is from the lower part of the body it is

---

[63] K xi, 310–11. Asclepiades, according to Celsus (iii.18.6) said that to let blood at the height of the fever was to commit murder.

[64] K x, 624–5; see also K vi, 263.   [65] K xi, 289–90; K x, 287ff.; K xv, 763ff.

[66] See above, p. 115, n. 65.   [67] K xi, 150.

[68] K xi, 168. Galen says that even a layman knows that venesection should be used in these conditions, but Erasistratus does not.

[69] K xi, 192–3.

[70] K xiv, 340–1; K xi, 299f. (above, pp. 91–2), a triumph over an Erasistratean haemophobe. Galen explains that venesection is necessary in order to evacuate the body before caustics are applied to the eyelids, to prevent them from becoming inflamed as a result of the treatment.

[71] K xviib, 81ff.

[72] K x, 930. Galen (K xi, 161–2; vii, 602–4) praises Hippocrates for venesecting a woman who was shivering, and might therefore be thought to require heating rather than cooling remedies (above, pp. 23–4); for further discussion see Chapter 2, K 161–2 and n. 29.

[73] K x, 658.   [74] K xi, 281.

revulsion, since the part to which the blood is attracted is far from the site of the haemorrhage. It is essential to apply the treatment on the side of the body on which the condition being treated is situated;[75] Galen says that revulsive venesection on the opposite side from the lesion is of no value.[76] To treat haemorrhage from the right nostril, cup the region of the liver; from the left, the region of the spleen; for bleeding from both nostrils, apply cups to both sides. This is revulsion, as seen also in the woman vomiting blood who was cured by the menstrual flow supervening.[77] Venesection, says Galen, can combine the functions of evacuation and revulsion.[78] As a general rule, a vein should be opened as far as possible from the spot where the blood collects in plethos.[79] Incipient inflammations should be revulsed in this way; when, however, they have become established, a part as near as possible to the affected one should be used. For example, incipient inflammations of the throat should be revulsed through the arm; when they have become established, through the sublingual veins.[80] Revulsive methods may be used, not only to subdue haemorrhage or to disperse plethos, but also to promote beneficial evacuations. When the haemorrhoidal flux is suppressed and it is desired to start it again, open a vein in the legs; this encourages the flux by drawing blood into the lower part of the body. To suppress the flux, however, draw blood from the arm.[81] In the same way, according to Galen, venesection in the arm checks the menstrual flow by revulsion,[82] and the Hippocratic writers, he says, recommended scarifying the ankles to bring on the menses.[83] Galen several times mentions specific sites for revulsive or derivative bloodletting. If there is plethos of the liver, use the right internal cubital vein, since it is directly connected with the vena cava.[84] For the mouth use the humeral vein, or as a second choice the median vein in the arm. For lesions of the occiput, open veins in the forehead and elbow. When the kidneys, bladder or pudenda are affected, open the popliteal veins.[85] To subdue inflammations of the uterus revulse through the arm, or cup the breasts; use the side corresponding to the side of the uterus that is affected. For diseases of the spleen, use the left arm; for the liver, the right.[86] Inflammations of the eye are treated by opening the humeral vein on the affected side.[87]

[75] K x, 315–16.   [76] K xi, 295–6.   [77] K x, 315–16; L 4, 542.
[78] K xi, 179.   [79] K xv, 149.   [80] K xi, 305.   [81] K xi, 307.
[82] K xi, 303. On the other hand Trousseau, *Lectures on clinical medicine* (1872), vol. v, p. 218, says: 'Bleeding from the arm . . . is a measure of immense potency [sc. to bring on the menses] and it is not unusual for the uterine flux to appear an hour after the bloodletting.'
[83] K xi, 283, 303.   [84] K x, 901.   [85] K x, 904.   [86] K xi, 91–2.   [87] K xi, 297

The question why Galen believed in revulsive bloodletting from the same side as the lesion is one of great interest, which as far as I know has not been previously considered. It cannot be answered without some preliminary consideration of his anatomy of the vascular system and that of his predecessors, and is therefore dealt with in a separate chapter.

This concludes the summary of Galen's indications for venesection. He had, however, certain principles which led him to perform, or not to perform, the operation where an indication for its use existed, and these will now be dealt with separately. Galen regards them as of great importance. They are, in brief, the strength of the patient's natural faculties; his physical type; his age; the previous history; the time of day, the season of the year, and the geographical region. The most important of these is the strength of the patient's powers or natural faculties; this discovery, together with that of the indication from the severity of the disease, he attributes to Hippocrates.[88] Galen mentions it repeatedly;[89] it may be estimated from the strength of the pulse,[90] which the physician must monitor carefully during the operation.[91] Some practitioners observe the principle of not letting blood after the fourth day of the illness, but this is wrong. If the patient is strong enough, he may be venesected even on the twentieth day; many patients, on the other hand, are already too weak by the second day to bear it.[92] The strength of the patient, again, is all that decides whether venesection should be used in old age; old patients can stand it if their powers are in good condition.[93] In general, however, its use should be confined to patients who are in the prime of life.[94] Galen never uses it in children less than fourteen years of age.[95] In commenting on the Hippocratic observation that venesection should be employed in acute diseases when the disease is severe and the patient strong, Galen asks whether these could be made the only rules for its use, and concludes that they could not, since they would not exclude the use of the remedy in children. Children, he says, are strong but should none the less not be venesected. This is because, owing to the warmth and dampness of their constitutions, their strength is readily broken down;[96] besides, they transpire readily and do not need the evacuation of phlebotomy.[97] Not only children, but some adults transpire well; this is a function of physical type. Those who are moderately lean

---

[88] K x, 286–7.
[89] K xi, 269, 277, 278, 281, 289–90, 291, 310. K x, 286ff., 565, 624, 777, 785. K xii, 523. K xv, 763ff.
[90] K xi, 291.   [91] K xi, 288.   [92] K xi, 308–10.   [93] K xi, 291.
[94] K x, 565; xv, 763ff.   [95] K xi, 290.   [96] K xv, 765.   [97] K x, 657–8.

and dark, with large veins, have much blood and benefit from venesection, but it should be undertaken with more caution in patients of the opposite kind, who have tender flesh and little blood and transpire readily.[98] Such patients are thin, sickly, and over-sensitive; the kind who should be bled freely are of more stocky build.[99]

Transpiration, according to Galen, is further affected by the crasis of the ambient air, and by the climate of the region. When these are hot and dry, transpiration, both through the breath and through sweating, is abundant; phlebotomy should therefore not be used at all, or with caution.[100] When, on the other hand, the climate and the air are damp and cold, sweating is reduced; venesection, in suitable patients, may then be more freely employed.[101] The season of the year must be taken into consideration, applying the same principles.[102] Galen offers a number of observations on transpiration in various species of animals.[103]

The patient's mode of life must also be considered. Those who are of temperate habits benefit from prophylactic venesection or purgation at the beginning of spring; this eliminates superfluous humours. Drunken and intemperate people, however, accumulate an excess of undigested humours, and do not benefit from such treatment; the physician should not undertake the management of such patients.[104]

Not only can bloodletting be undertaken, if strength permits, at any stage of the patient's disease, but it may also be used at any time of the day or night, in spite of the opinions of some physicians who let blood only between the second and the sixth hours of the day. Although Galen uses it at night,[105] he says the best time is early in the morning, preferably after the patient has been awake for an hour, and perhaps has taken a walk.[106]

Most of Galen's contraindications to venesection have already been mentioned. The modern Erasistrateans, Galen says, pay no attention to factors that ought to restrain them from venesection.[107] Apart from the all-important contraindication of weakness of the faculties, and those of childhood and old age, bodily constitution, state of the air and climate, which have been mentioned, venesection should be used with caution where there is an excess of crude humours,[108] and when fever is at its height;[109] it may, however, be used in continuous fevers if the faculties are in good condition. When, however, they are

---

[98] K xi, 290.   [99] K x, 624–7.   [100] K x, 658.   [101] K x, 624–7.
[102] K x, 930.   [103] K xi, 183–5.   [104] K xi, 272.   [105] K xi, 287–8.
[106] K xi, 310–11.   [107] K xi, 196.   [108] K xi, 282; K vi, 263.   [109] K xi, 282.

enfeebled and the humours are at the same time corrupted, extreme skill is necessary in employing the remedy.[110] In his commentary on *Regimen in Acute Diseases* Galen says that the author is quite wrong in employing venesection in hydrops, at least once the condition is established, if the patient is dyspnoeic; the danger of totally extinguishing the innate heat is too great.[111] It is also contraindicated in diarrhoea, lest the patient's powers be overthrown.[112] Galen agrees with Hippocrates that a pregnant woman must not be venesected;[113] this kills the foetus, Galen says, by depriving it of nourishment.[114]

As to the amount of the evacuation, Galen regards three cotyles[115] as a moderate one;[116] others recommend two.[117] Children who have reached the age of fourteen, if otherwise suitable for the operation, should not have more than one cotyle removed; a further half may be taken later.[118] Some patients cannot stand the removal of more than one and a half pounds of blood; others can tolerate six.[119] Ignorant people, says Galen, do not know that even very thin people can have too much blood. This is what was wrong with an anorexic woman who had not menstruated for eight months. On the first day he removed a pound and a half of blood, followed by a pound on the second and half a pound on the third, thus quickly restoring her to health. As she was from a prominent family he was subsequently consulted by many such patients, whom he cured in the same way.[120]

It is clear that Galen carefully judged the amount of blood to be removed; in appropriate cases, however, his treatment was often heroic. Evacuation to the point of fainting, he says – for example, six cotyles at once – is called for when there is a plethos of overheated blood. Patients treated in this way become cold, sweat, pass faeces, lose consciousness, and recover from their diseases; it is essential, however, to monitor the pulse carefully throughout the operation, or the patient may die. Galen knows of three doctors to whom this has happened.[121] Although copious venesection is the most effective means of extinguishing the flame of continuous fevers, it does great harm if wrongly applied; not only death but permanent incapacity may result.[122] Copious evacuations must be avoided, not only in very hot weather when loss by transpiration is great, but also when it is

[110] K x, 638–40.   [111] K xv, 892–3.   [112] K xv, 908.   [113] L 4, 542.
[114] K xviib, 821.   [115] About 850 ml, or one and a half Imperial pints.
[116] K xi, 174.   [117] K xi, 217–18.   [118] K xi, 290–1.
[119] K xi, 294. Six Roman pounds is about two litres, nearly half the total blood volume of a small adult.
[120] K xviib, 81ff.; perhaps the first account of anorexia nervosa in the literature.
[121] K xi, 288–9.   [122] K x, 637–8.

cold; this is because they chill the patient.[123] The great advantage of venesection as an evacuant is that it can be stopped at will.[124] Galen decides when to terminate it by observing the colour both of the issuing blood and of the patient's complexion, by his state of consciousness, by the cessation of flow from the vein, by the pulse, by collapse of the veins, and by sweating and vomiting.[125] The full amount to be taken is not necessarily removed at one operation; it is sometimes desirable to divide it among several, especially when there is an accumulation of crude humours.[126] This is known as epaphairesis (repeated removal), and the venesections may be performed on the same day or on successive ones.[127] If blood is let twice on the same day, the first evacuation should be the smaller.[128]

When Galen's practice of venesection is compared with that described in the Hippocratic corpus it is obvious that it is not only more extensive than that of the ancients, but also more codified. If the early physicians had rational rules for their practices, we do not know what they were; Galen, on the other hand, sometimes gives information about his. Little is known about the evolution of therapeutics between the Hippocratics and Galen, since most of the sources are lost. Some of the available ones, however, will be briefly considered in Chapter 9, after a chapter on Galen's relationship with the ancients in matters of applied vascular anatomy.

---

[123] K xi, 294.   [124] K xi, 286.   [125] K xi, 172, 217.
[126] K xi, 286.   [127] K xi, 297–8. See also Aretaeus vii.2.2. for epaphairesis.
[128] K vi, 296–7.

CHAPTER 8

Galen's revulsive treatment and vascular anatomy

In Galen's own time, some proponents of venesection believed that it was immaterial which vein was opened, since the same effect could equally well be obtained by using any of them;[1] others, Galen among them, thought that it made a great deal of difference which vessel was used.[2] Hippocrates and the most celebrated physicians, he says, were of this opinion also.[3] This is not an isolated opinion of Galen's; he expresses it in all three of his works on venesection, and he makes further mention of specific sites for bloodletting in the *De Sanitate Tuenda*,[4] the *De Methodo Medendi*,[5] *Ad Glauconem de Methodo Medendi*,[6] and his commentary on the *Aphorisms*.[7] Now Galen was an expert anatomist, and his view of the structure (as distinct from the function)[8] of the vascular system was, except in insignificant detail, that of the anatomist of today; yet he approved of practices of revulsive phlebotomy which, it would seem, must be quite inconsistent with such a view of vascular anatomy. To try to understand why he did this it will be necessary to summarise not only his own anatomical opinions, but also those of some of his predecessors, particularly those who offered clear accounts of the peripheral vessels.[9]

Since the vessels contain blood, and since blood has been a subject of interest to man from the earliest times,[10] we find some reference to

---

[1] K xi, 212, 218–20, 251.   [2] K xi, 178–9, 283, 284, 295–6.   [3] K xi, 169, 251.
[4] K vi, 297.
[5] K x, 316, 341, 904.   [6] K xi, 80–1, 91–3.   [7] K xviiia, 57.
[8] Cf. Harris: 'Galen's topographical scheme of the vascular system was reasonably correct; it was his physiological interpretation of the facts which was at fault' (p. 323).
[9] The late Hippocratic treatise *On the Heart* has not been considered, since it does not say enough about the peripheral vessels to be useful; nor the tract misnamed *Nature of Bones*, which says a good deal, but not in a comprehensible form. The same applies to *Epidemics* ii, for which see further Smith (1979), p. 149. For an account of vascular systems in the Hippocratic work *On Generation* and the rest of the Corpus see I. M. Lonie, *The Hippocratic treatises 'On Generation', 'On the Nature of the Child', 'Diseases IV'* (1981).
[10] A remarkable passage in the *Iliad*, which does not seem to have been noticed in this connection, implies that blood, which to the Hebrews was the life of the body (Lev. 17.11), was for Homer something that made man subject to death: 'And the immortal blood of the goddess flowed forth, ichor, such as flows in the blessed gods; for they

blood-vessels in the earliest Western literature. Homer describes how Antilochus, leaping on Thoon from behind, cut right through the vein that runs straight along the back till it arrives at the neck.[11] This vein appears in the earliest anatomical account we have in Greek, by a certain Syennesis; it has been preserved by Aristotle. Two principal veins are described. Each begins at the eye, runs along the eyebrow, along the back, past the lung, and under the breasts; the two veins cross, presumably somewhere in the epigastrium. The one coming from the left runs to the liver, kidney and testis; the one from the right to the spleen, kidney, testis and penis.

Aristotle next presents the system of Diogenes of Apollonia, which is more complicated; it may be summarised as follows: The two largest (or no. 1) vessels begin behind the ears and run down under the clavicles on either side of the spine. From these two veins, branches extend from the one on the right to the right-hand side of the body, and from the one on the left to the left side. The main branches of these vessels, from the top down, are a pair going through the lower part of the axilla to the arm and down to the thumb; the left branch is called the splenetic, the right the hepatic vein. These vessels, in spite of their names, do not communicate directly with their corresponding organs; they are perhaps named according to their uses in venesection. A little further down, each no. 1 vessel communicates with the heart. Next, the right vessel sends a branch to the liver, the left to the spleen and left kidney. At the groin each vessel forks and sends a double supply to the leg on the corresponding side.

The next or no. 2 pair start in the neck and go down into the chest; branches accompany the splenetic and hepatic veins to the arms, 'below the shoulder-blades and towards the hands'. These are the vessels from which doctors let blood when pain is felt under the skin (unfortunately Diogenes does not say where), whereas for pain in the bowels they open the splenetic and hepatic veins. The no. 2 veins also supply the region below the breasts.

The no. 3 pair run on either side of the spinal marrow to the testes. No. 4 are called the spermatic vessels; they run just under the skin to the kidneys, ending in the testes or uterus according to sex. Diogenes seems to say that pairs 3 and 4 are branches of the large veins, presumably no. 1; it is not clear where they originate. Lastly there are the vessels of the stomach; they are broad at first, but

do not eat bread, nor do they drink flashing wine, and therefore they are bloodless and are called immortals' (*Il.* v.339–42). This idea is perhaps supported by the similarity of the words βροτός, mortal, and βρότος, gore.
[11] *Il.* xiii.545–7.

become narrower as they cross over to the opposite side of the body.[12]

If we exclude these stomach veins from consideration – and they would not be accessible to venesectionists in any case – we have here a system of paired vessels providing an independent venous supply to the left and right halves of the body. A similar, but simpler, double system is found in the Hippocratic work *On the Sacred Disease*, the production of a pneumatist. The brain is in two halves; from it extend two chief veins, one going to the liver and the other to the spleen. The one to the liver is the larger; in its lower part it is called the hollow vein. Above the liver it communicates with the heart and the right arm, and then leads upwards under the clavicle into the neck, where it can be seen; it supplies the brain, eye, ear and nostril on the right side. Below the liver it extends down to the right foot. On the left side there is a similar but more slender vein, passing in the same way through the spleen.[13] The vein on the right appears to be the vena cava, but it supplies the right side of the body only and does not bifurcate in the lower abdomen. The main supplies to the two sides of the body are still independent.

Next we have the description of the veins given in the Hippocratic tract *Nature of Man*. Galen refers to this work in his book *On the Natural Faculties*, describing it as a very fine work by Hippocrates himself.[14] He does not consider the account of the veins to be by him, however, nor by his son-in-law Polybus to whom Aristotle attributes it.[15] There are four main pairs of veins. The no. 1 pair start in the head, and go straight down on either side of the spine to supply the legs; they lie on the outer side of the ankles and extend to the feet. Venesection for pain in the back and loins, says the author, should therefore be performed behind the knee or at the outer side of the ankle. The no. 2 pair are the jugulars; they start at the ears, run down the spine like the first pair, supply the testes, run on the inner side of the thigh to the popliteal fossa, and thence via the inner side of the ankle to the feet. So for pain in the loins and testes, bleeding should be performed behind the knee or on the inside of the ankle. The third pair of veins start at the temples and go down through the neck to the lungs, where they cross; the one that started on the right then supplies

---

[12] Aristotle, *Hist. An.* 3.2. Harris (pp. 456–9) provides diagrams of some of the ancient systems. This has not been done here because of the danger of giving an impression of precision that is lacking in the original schemes.

[13] L 6, 366.   [14] K II, 132.

[15] K v, 529. Galen says that only the first part of this work is genuine (K xv, 9–10, 108). The true Hippocratic doctrine, he says, can be found in *Epidemics* II and in *Nutriment* (K v, 529). There is, however, no detailed account of veins in *Nutriment* as we have it, while the passage in *Epidemics* II (L 5, 120–4) is almost incomprehensible.

the spleen and left kidney, the other the liver and right kidney, and finally they unite at the anus. The no. 4 veins begin at the eyes, go down the neck and into the arm via its upper part (this is probably the cephalic vein of modern anatomists, though it does not connect with the eyes), down to the hand where they loop back and return to the axilla whence they go to the ribs, the right-hand vein supplying the liver and the left the spleen; thence they go to the genitalia. We have here a direct connection between a vein in the left arm and the spleen, and between one in the right arm and the liver, of the kind expected from the naming of the arm veins in the system of Diogenes; it is tempting to conjecture that the names splenetic and hepatic in Diogenes' account, as we have it, might originate from a gloss made by someone who was familiar with the system described in *Nature of Man*. The author of *Nature of Man* tells us further that there are veins of all kinds extending from the belly to the rest of the body, through which nourishment is distributed to it. Veins also lead from the main veins to the belly and the rest of the body, both from the outside and the inside, communicating with one another in both directions. His general rule for venesection follows: one should open a vein as far as possible from the place where the pain is felt and the blood collects, so that the change will be least violent and the habit of the blood of collecting in the affected part will be changed.[16] Galen comments on this rule,[17] observing that the author should distinguish between incipient and established lesions.

This system, like those described earlier, is basically double, though the author adds that there are numerous intercommunications between the principal veins. In the Hippocratic work *Airs, Waters, Places* the author, discussing the Scythians, remarks that they are in the habit of opening the veins behind the ears, after which they fall asleep; when they wake they find themselves impotent. 'For alongside the ears there are veins which, if one should cut them, make them impotent, and it seems to me that these are the veins they cut.'[18] These would appear to be the no. 2 veins of *Nature of Man*, which start behind the ear and supply the testes on their way to the feet, and the veins in *On Places in Man* (see below) that lead to sterility when cut.[19] The description in *The Sacred Disease* includes no vein supplying the genitals, which perhaps makes it unlikely that *Airs, Waters, Places* and *The Sacred Disease* are by the same author, as some have thought possible. The author of *Regimen in Acute Diseases*, who recommends bleeding from what seems to be the no. 4 vein of *Nature of Man* for

---

[16] L 6, 58–60.   [17] K xv, 149–50; see also K xi, 305.   [18] L 2, 78.
[19] For an explanation of this effect, see the Hippocratic work *Generation* (L 7, 472–4).

pains in the chest, would appear also to accept this view of vascular anatomy.[20]

The tract *On Places in Man* offers another system. Leaving out, as irrelevant to our subject, the author's interesting account of the temporal arteries, we come to the following system of principal veins. The first pair pass through the neck, down the spine, and end in the kidneys; they also connect with the testes. Disease of these veins leads to haematuria. The second pair lead from the crown of the head to the shoulders; they are called the shoulder veins (ὠμαῖαι). A third pair also start from the top of the head, travel alongside the ears, down the front of the neck on each side, and join to form the hollow vein, which runs between the trachea and the oesophagus; it passes through the heart and diaphragm and forks to supply each leg, the two branches running down the inner side of the leg and ankle to the foot. These, says the author, are the veins that make a person sterile if they are cut. Another branch of the hollow vein goes to the left flank and chest and to the spleen, connecting with the shoulder vein;[21] there is a similar branch on the right side. 'All the veins communicate and flow into one another' says the author.[22]

We have here a system that is partially double (the no. 1 and 2 veins) and partially single. The author has the right idea of the vena cava as a single vessel which branches in the lower abdomen to supply both legs. There is, as before, a shoulder vein (the modern cephalic) which comes, not from the eyes this time, but from the top of the head; it is joined by a branch of the vena cava which passes through the liver on the right, and through the spleen on the left. The author does not make it clear where this union takes place; if it is in the arm, as Littré interpreted it, we have a hepatic and a splenetic vein as in Diogenes and *Nature of Man*. The anatomy shows a distinct advance in the lower part of the body, and again there are communications between the veins mentioned.

When Aristotle has quoted Syennesis, Diogenes, and the author of *Nature of Man* on the venous system, he says that they are all wrong, since they place the origin of the blood vessels in the head, whereas in fact they originate in the heart. He then gives his own account of the vessels at some length. The essential points for the present argument are as follows. Above the heart the great vein divides into two, and

[20] L 2, 272.
[21] Littré translates to make this vein join the shoulder vein at the bend of the elbow, and says it is opened in disease of the spleen. I follow the interpretation of Harris (p. 47) which seems to represent the Greek more accurately; but the passage is somewhat obscure.
[22] L 6, 280–2.

from each branch arise the jugular and subclavian veins (this is correct). The jugulars run upwards to the ears, where, he says, they divide into two; one branch loops back and runs down the neck again into the arm, joining the continuation of the subclavian vein at the bend of the elbow. This is clearly the modern cephalic vein, which joins the basilic by the median cubital; its origin, however, is quite wrong. The other branch, says Aristotle, terminates in the hand and the fingers; it is not clear what this means, unless he thinks there is another vein running down the arm. Below the heart the vena cava runs down and divides in the lower abdomen to supply the legs. It provides on its way, however, a branch to the liver which continues to the right arm, meeting the two veins already mentioned at the bend of the elbow; the same thing happens on the left side with a branch through the spleen. The one in the right arm, says Aristotle, is opened when patients have pains in the region of the liver.[23]

This is an advance in that the entire system is now single, but the fictions of a cephalic vein originating in the head (in fact it branches from the subclavian vein) and of special hepatic and splenetic veins in the arms are preserved.

All the systems hitherto mentioned provide some excuse for the practice of letting blood from a particular vein when some particular part of the body is affected. In particular, those postulating independent venous supplies to the two halves of the body provide the justification for revulsive venesection on the side of the lesion, and explain why haemorrhages that occur naturally may be thought beneficial to lesions on the same side of the body. Even the systems, like Aristotle's, that are more or less correct in the lower part of the body, still provide a reason for such practices as opening the cephalic vein on the affected side in ophthalmia, and a vein in the right elbow when the liver is affected, but on the left for diseases of the spleen. Galen, as has been shown, repeatedly recommends such practices; does his own anatomy of the vascular system support his methods?

No one with any knowledge of anatomy who comes to Galen's anatomical works after reading the accounts of the vascular system described above can fail to notice a profound difference. Although his work *On the Anatomy of the Veins and Arteries* is based on dissections of monkeys, very little change would be necessary to make it apply accurately to the anatomy of man, with which, in any case, Galen had some considerable acquaintance. Galen is an anatomist; the others, even the great Aristotle, are writers of fiction. The following summary of Galen's views concerns only the main features of the veins that are

[23] *Hist. An.* 3.3–4.

important for venesection; even in his synopses, such as the work mentioned, he refers to a great number of other vessels in the most careful detail.

He describes correctly the bifurcation of the superior vena cava to form what are now called the innominate veins, and the origin of the internal jugular from them. (A modern anatomist, of course, describes the veins in the reverse direction, from the periphery to the heart.) The trunks continue through the axilla and down the arms (modern basilic vein), and at the bend of the elbow they meet, via the median cubital, the cephalic veins, which he says arise from a branch of the subclavian, the external jugular vein; this is the vein that Galen describes as encircling the clavicle. In man the cephalic usually branches directly from the subclavian, but Galen's arrangement, which may well be the normal one in monkeys, is sanctioned in man by Gray: 'Sometimes it (the cephalic vein) communicates with the external jugular vein by a branch which ascends in front of the clavicle.'[24] At the bend of the elbow the basilic and cephalic are connected by the short median cubital vein, thus providing the three veins at the elbow frequently mentioned by Galen as sites for venesection. Below the heart Galen correctly describes the inferior vena cava, and he has no arm veins directly connected with the liver or spleen.[25]

Can Galen justify his practice on the basis of his anatomy? His most convincing argument would probably apply to the cephalic vein (Galen's humeral vein) in diseases of the eye on the same side of the body. As previously mentioned, Galen believes that this vein arises, not from the subclavian itself, but from one of its branches, the external jugular;[26] and it is perfectly true that this vein drains (in the modern terminology; Galen would say 'nourishes') the corresponding side of the face. But even in Galen's monkeys the origin of the cephalic must be very near the subclavian. With the veins in the arm, however, Galen is quite illogical. For plethos of the liver, he says, use the inner vein (i.e. the basilic) at the right elbow, since it is directly connected with the vena cava.[27] So it is; but the same applies to the corresponding vein in the left arm, except that the vena cava is a little nearer to the right-hand vein by virtue of its situation slightly to the right of the midline. It applies, too, to the cephalic vein; both the cephalic and the basilic, as Galen knew very well, have their origin in or very near the subclavian, and it should make no difference at all whether one opened the cephalic, the basilic or the median cubital vein at the elbow. On his principle, indeed, that one should open a vein as far as

[24] *Gray's Anatomy, descriptive and applied,* 28th ed. (1945) p. 821.   [25] K II, 786–801.
[26] K II, 800.   [27] K x, 901.

possible from the spot where the blood collects,[28] it would surely be more logical to open the *left* cubital veins for inflammations of the liver, at least in their early stages, thus revulsing the plethos to the opposite side of the body. Galen's insistence that the vein on the right must be used is an anachronism from the days when there was a special hepatic vein in the right arm; perhaps the divine Hippocrates believed it. He has the same views, which are equally without foundation, about using the veins of the left arm when the spleen is affected.[29] It seems impossible to avoid the conclusion that his practice is based on a theory which he knows to be discredited.[30] He is very definite, however, about the importance of using the correct side. The beneficial effect of haemorrhages on the same side as the lesion, he says, can be observed daily in patients; Hippocrates was the first to notice and describe them, observing that contralateral haemorrhages were deleterious.[31] If you revulse on the same side as the lesion, says Galen, the patient's relief will be quickly evident; if you open a vein on the opposite side it does not help at all. For a haemorrhage from the left nostril one should cup the left hypochondrium, not the right;[32] on the system of Diogenes this would make good sense, but it seems to make none at all on Galen's. It cannot be argued that these are early opinions, which Galen revised as his knowledge of anatomy increased; they are from his third book on venesection, one of the last of his works.

Galen does, in fact, say that in his time some physicians believed that it made no difference which vein was opened, whereas others, with the authority of Hippocrates, held that it was of the utmost importance to use the appropriate one.[33] Galen is a Hippocratist, and it would be tempting to assume that his reverence for the father of medicine might explain the discrepancies between his anatomy and his practice. It is clear enough that Galen was prepared to attribute certain parts of certain works in the Corpus to Hippocrates himself – as has already been shown for parts of the *Appendix* to *Regimen in Acute Diseases* – and to reject other parts of the same works because he does not agree with the opinions expressed in them. Wilamowitz is said to have described Hippocrates as a name without writings; Galen, who may well have had no more facts at his disposal, constructed for himself a Hippocrates who agreed with Galen, and endowed the opinions of this fictitious being with almost divine authority. One

---

[28] K xv, 149–50.   [29] K xi, 91–2.

[30] This, however, may be the result of looking at Galen from the point of view of a modern; for an attempt to understand his own outlook, see the following chapter.

[31] L 5, 652–4, 554. See also L 3, 120; L 5, 146.   [32] K xi, 295–6.

[33] K xi, 212, 218–20, 251.

might alternatively postulate that in Galen's time the whole Corpus had, for some people at least, something of the authority which, till recently, the Bible had for the more fundamentalist sects; he accepted its authority as final, merely because it existed, without enquiring into its origins.[34] This would explain very well why Galen, if he was a fundamentalist, still believed in revulsion on the affected side although he knew that anatomy did not support its use; he would have been in the same position as the nineteenth-century man brought up to take everything in the book of Genesis literally, when confronted with the fossil record. But it has already been shown that Galen is not a fundamentalist where the Corpus is concerned; he picks and chooses, and this is certainly not a mark of the fundamentalist, but rather of the devotee of the Higher Criticism. Why, then, does he believe things that must be seen to be false by any unprejudiced observer today? It might of course be argued that practices such as bleeding from the right arm in diseases of the liver were so entrenched by tradition that no practitioner would risk his reputation by deviating from them.[35] As will be shown later, however, there was no such tradition; and this in any case would not account for Galen's belief in the Hippocratic doctrine of the efficacy of naturally occurring haemorrhages, provided they were on the same side of the body as the lesion. Simple observation of patients should have convinced him that this was false; yet it was believed implicitly by a practitioner of great ability and enormous experience and industry. For some reason he was not an unprejudiced observer. It has already been shown that, for Galen, the Hippocratic corpus could not claim divine inspiration in toto, and he clearly did not accept the whole of it as revealed truth. If he did not agree with a particular part of the Corpus, all he had to say was that it was not a genuine utterance of Hippocrates. We have, too, his own statement that in his time certain practitioners did not accept his

[34] For the possible existence of such ideas in antiquity see Smith (1979), p. 178.

[35] It is regarded as unethical today to conduct a clinical trial, if any risk is involved, with a drug that is probably ineffective; there must be a reasonable chance of benefit to patients if the test is to be justified. Since venesection is a remedy not without danger, it might be argued that no one would ever have tried the effect of letting blood from the left arm in diseases of the liver, once the tradition of using the right had become established; the damage to the doctor's reputation would be too great if the patient did not do well. A passage from Celsus (Prooem. 50) is relevant here: 'I think that nothing was tried because no one was prepared to risk an experiment on a distinguished patient, for fear that, if he did not save her, it might appear that he had killed her.' Edelstein has convincingly shown how important reputation was to the ancient practitioner; see his essay on 'Hippocratic prognosis' in *Ancient medicine: selected papers of Ludwig Edelstein* (1967) pp. 65ff. One must admire the courage of Erasistratus, who refused altogether to use venesection in the face of almost all ancient tradition and practice. Whether he was altogether right in doing this will be considered in a later chapter.

decided views; they thought that any vein would do. But was there a tradition, and were these dissenting doctors an insignificant group of heretics, obstinately resisting the known truth? Galen is such a contentious author that his own works cannot be relied on to answer this, and independent sources must be examined. Unfortunately most of the works between the last of the Hippocratic authors and Galen's own time are lost; some that have survived, however, will be briefly considered in the following chapter.

CHAPTER 9

The testimony of other writers and the validity of Galen's opinions on sites for venesection

No attempt at an exhaustive analysis of the writers between Hippocrates and Galen will be made here. Only a few will be considered; the aim is merely to illustrate the divergent opinions that were prevalent.

Whether or not Celsus was himself a physician, and whether his work is his own or a translation of a lost Greek original, it is of the greatest value in reconstructing medical opinion between the Hippocratic writers and Galen. In addition to many incidental references he devotes a chapter to venesection, which opens with the significant remark: 'It is not new to let blood by cutting a vein; but that there is hardly any disease in which blood is not let, is new.'[1] This is, in effect, Galen's indication from the severity of the disease, regardless of its nature; his primary indication for bloodletting is the presence, or indeed only the expectation, of any severe disease whatsoever.[2] According to Celsus this was in his time – some two centuries before Galen, unless he is reproducing an earlier work – a new concept. It cannot be Hippocratic, since Celsus describes Hippocrates as 'the most ancient author'.[3] As we have seen, the idea appears in the Corpus only in the *Appendix* to *Regimen in Acute Diseases*, which most scholars think spurious, although Galen says that this particular statement is good Hippocratic doctrine; this does not apply, however, to everything else in the treatise.[4] It has already been shown that the Hippocratic writers used venesection far less extensively than Galen did, though Galen would like us to think otherwise; Celsus confirms this opinion. His practice in using the remedy in almost all diseases is already in agreement with Galen's later methods; in other respects, however, it differs notably.

Hippocrates, as already mentioned, forbade venesection in pregnancy,[5] and Galen agrees;[6] Celsus, however, holds that it may be used in pregnant women, and in patients of any age whatsoever, as long as strength permits.[7] Hippocrates has already been superseded. 'Later

---

[1] Celsus II.10.1.   [2] K xi, 150; see above, p. 17.   [3] Celsus, Prooem. 66.
[4] See above, p. 115, n. 65.
[5] L 4, 542.   [6] K xviib, 821.   [7] Celsus II.10.1–2.

practice however showed that there is nothing final in this . . . for it is
the patient's strength that is important, not age, nor whether there is
pregnancy.'[8] This is a most significant remark, showing as it does that
there was nothing sacrosanct about the Corpus; practice had shown
that it was wrong, and new methods were introduced. Galen never
used venesection in children under the age of fourteen, but this was
evidently not a universally observed prohibition. 'A strong child, or a
robust old man, or a healthy pregnant woman may be safely treated'[9]
(sc. by venesection), says Celsus. He makes it clear that this too is a
new practice. 'It is not an old practice for the same to be used in
children, in the aged, and also in pregnant women.'[10] Venesection
may be necessary in fever and inflammatory conditions; in severe
pain; in contusion of the viscera, in patients with a bad bodily habitus,
and in all acute diseases. Sometimes bloodletting is urgently called for
although the patient is too weak to bear it safely; such patients must
be venesected boldly, after explaining the risks.[11]

The second or third day of the illness, according to Celsus, is better
than the first for venesection, since the food taken before the illness
will by then have been digested. Venesection may be necessary on the
first day, but is never of service after the fourth, since then it merely
weakens without restoring the body to health.[12] This, again, is at
variance with Galen's practice; he was prepared to let blood even on
the twentieth day if the patient's strength permitted.[13] Celsus is far
less exacting than Galen on the choice of sites for venesection. Where
the disease affects the whole body the arm should be used, but no side
is specified; for localised lesions, a vein as near as possible to the site
of the lesion should be opened. Celsus says he is well aware that some
remove blood from a vein as far as possible from the affected part, in
order to divert the course of the material of the disease; but this, he
says, is wrong. Venesection removes blood from the nearest parts
first.[14] He admits that it can be used revulsively to stop bleeding, but
does not specify which vein should be opened: 'The flow of blood
from an unwanted place stops, when something is applied to prevent
it, if another way of escape for the blood is provided.'[15] Experience
has shown, however, that the arm should be used for venesection
when the head has been injured. When the shoulder or arm is
affected, blood should be taken from the opposite arm; this is not for
reasons of vascular anatomy, but simply because the injured arm is
more liable to the complications of phlebotomy than the sound one

---

[8] Celsus II.10.2.   [9] Celsus II.10.3.   [10] Celsus II.10.1.   [11] Celsus II.10.6–8.
[12] Celsus II.10.9–10.   [13] K XI, 308–10.   [14] Celsus II.10.12–13.
[15] Celsus II.10.14.

is.[16] Elsewhere Celsus recommends venesection from the arm where there is suppression of the menses;[17] this in direct contradiction of Galen, who lets blood from the lower parts in amenorrhoea. To take it from the arm, he says, suppresses the flow.[18] Celsus scarifies and cups the groins in menorrhagia;[19] Galen would use the upper parts of the body. Celsus agrees with the ancients, and with Galen, that the haemorrhoidal flux is a desirable evacuation.[20] Except in the one place mentioned, however, he nowhere specifies the artificial removal of blood from a particular side of the body for a particular condition. In disease of the liver, he says, venesection should be used, but no side is specified.[21]

Aretaeus[22] wrote somewhat later; he was probably a contemporary of Galen. For phrenitis, he says, bleed from the arm, using particularly the middle vein; the side is not mentioned.[23] When the lesion is in the head, do not take blood from the arm; he recommends bloodletting, but does not say from where.[24] In lethargy which is not secondary to other conditions, but may be associated with plethora, bleed from the elbow.[25] Phlebotomy, 'a great remedy for a great disease', is the principal remedy in apoplexy, but it is not easy to determine the amount of blood to take; too little is ineffective, while too much is fatal.[26] An elbow vein should be used, preferably the left; in lesser attacks use the unaffected side. The elbow is also used in tetanus; the side is not mentioned.[27] In synanche the arm is again recommended, with evacuation pushed to the point of loss of consciousness.[28] Copious evacuation from the elbow is also recommended in inflammation of the uvula.[29] In pleurisy, venesection must be undertaken without delay, using the elbow on the opposite side from the lesion, because it is as far as possible from the affected part.[30] Galen, in his third work on venesection, recommends the opposite course: 'In the pleurisies, phlebotomy on the affected side often shows the most obvious benefit, while taking blood from the other arm leads to indefinite or delayed results.'[31] In peripneumonia Aretaeus recommends that both arms be used, in order to revulse humours from both sides of the lungs, but not to the extent of the patient fainting, since this aggravates the suffocation. When some relief has been obtained, stop the flow, and repeat the treatment later; for the venesection removes the exciting causes if they are in the blood, whereas if phlegm

---

[16] Celsus II.10.14.   [17] Celsus IV.27.1D.   [18] K XI, 307.   [19] Celsus IV.27.1D.
[20] Celsus VI.18.9.   [21] Celsus IV.15.2.
[22] References to Aretaeus are to the edition of C. Hude, Berlin 1958.
[23] Aretaeus V.1.4.   [24] Aretaeus V.1.6.   [25] Aretaeus V.2.3.
[26] Aretaeus V.4.1–2.   [27] Aretaeus V.6.2.   [28] Aretaeus V.7.2.
[29] Aretaeus V.8.3.   [30] Aretaeus V.10.1–2.   [31] K XI, 297.

or other humours are involved, the emptying of the veins widens the field (χώρα) of the lungs for the passage of breath.[32] Where blood is being brought up, either by coughing or by vomiting, venesection must be used; the middle vein at the elbow is the preferred site for diseases of all the vital organs. Both the modern basilic and median cubital veins, Aretaeus says, are connected with the humeral (modern cephalic), so that the basilic is no better than the median, although ignorant people have connected it with the stomach and liver. Again, in diseases of the spleen, some physicians recommend a vein in the left hand, between the little and ring fingers, which they believe to connect with the spleen; but, says Aretaeus, this vein is a branch of those at the elbow, and it is better to open it there, where the vessels are larger.[33] Galen recommends both the vein in the hand and at the elbow for diseases of the spleen.[34]

Aretaeus recommends that intestinal obstruction should be treated by venesection if it is due to inflammation; blood should be removed copiously from a vein at the elbow. It may be carried to loss of consciousness, for the pain is so severe that the patient longs to die, and although it is not proper for the responsible practitioner to engage in euthanasia, he can at least relieve pain by a temporary loss of sensibility.[35] For disease of the liver, blood should be abstracted in frequent, though not large, amounts; a particular arm is not specified.[36] Leeches are recommended in some cases,[37] as also for the coeliac disease.[38] Large quantities of blood may be removed in disease of the large arteries,[39] of the kidneys,[40] and in satyriasis, since, says Aretaeus, it is the excess of blood that inflames the heat and lust.[41] Both the elbow and the ankle should be used, as also, together with both arms, in elephantiasis.[42] Like the Hippocratic writers, Aretaeus recommends bleeding from the lower limbs in diseases of the uterus.[43] For headache, use the elbow.[44] It has already been shown that Aretaeus does not distinguish between one arm vein and another. The straight vein of the forehead is also recommended.[45] The only reference I can find in Aretaeus to venesection on the affected side concerns

---

[32] Aretaeus vi.1.1.   [33] Aretaeus vi.2.1–4.   [34] K xi, 296–7.

[35] Aretaeus vi.5.1; the text, however, is uncertain here. According to Caelius Aurelianus, some physicians deliberately bled insane patients to death, taking blood from both arms (*CD* i.174).

[36] Aretaeus vi.6.2.

[37] Aretaeus vi.6.3. Galen apparently does not use leeches therapeutically, unless the short work *De Hirudinibus* (K xi, 317–22) is genuine; I think it is not. Galen mentions them in another context at K viii, 265 and 266.

[38] Aretaeus viii.7.3.   [39] Aretaeus vi.7.1–2.   [40] Aretaeus vi.8.3.

[41] Aretaeus vi.11.2.   [42] Aretaeus viii.13.3.   [43] Aretaeus vi.10.3.

[44] Aretaeus vii.2.1.   [45] Aretaeus vii.2.2–3.

melancholia; he recommends bleeding from the right elbow, to obtain a flow from the liver, which is the source of the blood and the origin of the bile, both of which provide nourishment for melancholy.[46]

It is clear that Aretaeus, like Galen, is a far more copious venesectionist than the Hippocratic authors. He is, however, far less committed than Galen is to the use of specific sites for venesection, and his views on applied anatomy are somewhat more enlightened, though he still believes in using the right arm in disease of the liver. Generally he venesects in the arm, without specifying the side. It is interesting to note that, like the Erasistrateans, he also recommends bandaging the limbs.[47] But, like Galen, he uses bloodletting and gives food in acute diseases, such as pleurisy.[48]

The observations of Antyllus (second century AD) as preserved by Oribasius, chiefly concern practical methods rather than principles. There are some useful extracts from Antyllus' lost book *On Evacuant Remedies*, including a good deal on local sites for venesection but very little mention of a particular side of the body. Antyllus, in fact, seems to favour particular veins, when they are suitable for incision, often without specifying the diseases for which they should be opened. To bleed from the forehead, use the straight vein in its upper part, where it divides in the shape of a Y. Behind the ears, the vein lying opposite to the cartilage should be used. Under the tongue, if we do not open both sides, we should use the larger vein, which is on the right; this seems to be Antyllus' only surviving reference to using a vein on a particular side of the body, and makes no mention of the situation of the lesion for which the venesection is undertaken. On the back of the hand the vein to open is the one between the middle and ring fingers. In the ham use the most central vein; at the ankle the inner; if there is only one in front and one behind, the front one. Owing, however, to the smallness of the veins we cannot always open the one we would like to. At the elbow any available vein may be used, but where there is a choice, Antyllus offers certain rules. In patients who need repeated evacuations or vigorous depletion use the middle vein; in those, however, in need of change and variety, such as epileptics, madmen and sufferers from scotomata, the lower (basilic) vein should be opened. This vein, according to Antyllus, is like an artery. He provides interesting practical details of the operation.[49]

Antyllus observes that where copious evacuation is required a large incision should be made, whereas if the aim is to divert the blood, as in

---

[46] Aretaeus VII.5.1–2.   [47] E.g. Aretaeus VI.10.3; VII.3.6.   [48] Aretaeus V.10.3–4.
[49] *Oribasii collectionum medicarum reliquiae*, ed. J. Raeder (1928), vol. I, p. 208.

patients who are bringing it up or bleeding from some part of the body, it should be very small. The patient's condition itself, he says, is evacuating him; he does not need further evacuation, but revulsion. The blood should be allowed to flow for a long time from the small incision. He makes no mention of the side of the body from which revulsion should take place.[50]

Although Caelius Aurelianus probably wrote in the fifth century, his work sets forth the opinions of Soranus, the leader of the Methodist sect in the first half of the second century AD, and also mentions those of many other practitioners. It is thus an extremely valuable source. There are numerous references to venesection, but relatively little mention of bleeding from a particular part or side of the body, and where there is, Caelius is often in disagreement with Galen. In pleurisy, he says, venesection should be performed on the side opposite to the one affected, 'for a reason we have often stated'.[51] He tells us elsewhere what this reason is. If headache is generalised, use either arm; but if it is unilateral, use the opposite arm, so that the disturbance occasioned by the treatment may be kept as far away as possible from the part affected.[52] This is a general principle of Soranus's, leading him not to take blood from the affected part. Themison used to bleed from arms and legs that were the seat of pain; Soranus condemns this, on the grounds that such treatment leads to a flow of blood to the venesected part, which may even exceed in quantity the amount withdrawn; the last state of the part is thus worse than the first, and by virtue of the disease in it the ill effects of such a concourse of humour are likely to be worse than they would be in an unaffected part.[53] Themison, again, bled from parts affected by motor

---

[50] Ibid. p. 212. On the previous page Antyllus describes the operation of bleeding from the forehead, corners of the eyes, and sublingual veins. To make these veins prominent a tourniquet is put round the neck, and the patient, to avoid suffocation, puts his hand or thumb inside the tourniquet below his chin. Antyllus helpfully explains that if he is paralysed an assistant, standing alongside, can literally lend a hand.

[51] Caelius, *AD* II.105.

[52] Caelius, *CD* I.11. Celsus (II.10.14) agrees; but see also II.10.12–13.

[53] Caelius, *CD* I.140–1; *AD* I.182. In the same way, it is wrong to apply leeches to the head for headache, as Themison, misguidedly following Asclepiades, used to do; it leads only to worse congestion. There are numerous references to the therapeutic use of leeches in Caelius' book; cf. Galen, who apparently never used them.

Themison (c. 31 BC–AD 14) was a pupil of Asclepiades, whose materialist ideas he developed to found the Methodist sect. The Methodists took a highly simplified view of medicine; there were only two basic pathological conditions, constriction and relaxation, and the aim of treatment was to loosen what was constricted, and to constrict what was loosened. Soranus of Ephesus practised in Rome in the second century, but before Galen's time; he is perhaps the only Methodist of whom Galen speaks with respect. His system has been preserved in the works of Caelius Aurelianus.

paralysis, as long as sensation was intact; Caelius says that this should be avoided, as it might injure them.[54]

Diocles, according to Caelius, took blood from patients with intestinal obstruction from the inner vein of the right arm, when the patient was young and strong. But this, says Caelius, is wrong; venesection may be used in patients of any age if strength permits, and instead of the right interior vein the left exterior may be more appropriate.[55] Again, Hippocrates recommends bloodletting from the internal arm vein (Caelius does not mention that he added 'on the affected side') in pleurisy, but only when the pain is extending upwards.[56] Soranus disagrees; any vein will do, and it is of no importance whether the pain extends upwards or downwards. To carry the evacuation to loss of consciousness, as Hippocrates recommended here, is very dangerous according to Soranus.[57] Themison, however, was not concerned about loss of consciousness; he let blood copiously from various parts of the body, including the ankles and arms,[58] and from the nostrils, ears and corners of the eyes for dysentery, a useless procedure according to Caelius.[59] Both arms, according to Soranus, should not be used, since this leads to fainting.[60] Diocles, however, bled full-blooded patients with synanche from both arms, while those with little blood were merely scarified. Caelius uses only one arm – he does not say which – and his only criterion is the patient's strength.[61]

In diseases of the liver and spleen, bleeding from the affected part is mentioned. Some physicians, such as Apollonius of Citium, rejected venesection altogether in diseases of the spleen; others approved of it, using the left arm, while the right was employed in diseases of the liver. Others, again, used the two ankles in the same way. These, says Caelius, are conflicting opinions; the fact is that such practitioners use veins that are easy to open, but not when they are swollen, since venesection should be performed far from the affected parts to avoid harm to them.[62] Diocles venesected the right arm in diseases of the liver, and used the remedy – the side is not stated – also in disease of the spleen.[63] Praxagoras let blood in diseases of both organs; Caelius says nothing about the side.[64] Themison was one of those who bled from the ankles on the affected side in these conditions; he also cauterised the liver and spleen. But his ideas about using the affected side, says Caelius, are impudent and

---

[54] Caelius, *CD* II.57.   [55] Caelius, *AD* III.159–61.   [56] L 2, 458–60.
[57] Caelius, *AD* II.114–22. Soranus has none of Galen's reverence for Hippocrates, but he attributes the *Appendix* to *Regimen in Acute Diseases* to him.
[58] Caelius, *CD* I.142.   [59] Caelius, *CD* IV.91.   [60] Caelius, *CD* I.174.
[61] Caelius, *AD* III.31.   [62] Caelius, *CD* III.56.   [63] Caelius, *CD* III.62.
[64] Caelius, *CD* III.64.

futile.[65] In diseases of the liver Erasistratus, according to Caelius, laid bare the organ and packed it round with drugs;[66] others suggested excision of the diseased spleen, but probably never performed it.[67]

In sciatica, too, some physicians opened a vein at the ankle or knee on the affected side, but Caelius says that this only increases the congestion and heaviness of the parts, since as soon as they are emptied they attract a flow of matter to themselves.[68]

Asclepiades, says Caelius, used venesection only where there was pain. He did not let blood at the onset of peripneumonia, saying that only thin and watery blood would escape; but Caelius maintains that the appearance of the blood is of no importance, and that venesection is useful in some patients who have no pain.[69] Themison also used the colour of the blood as an indication for stopping the flow.[70] Asclepiades bled from multiple sites in synanche: the forehead, corners of the eyes, sublingual veins and the arm. In severe cases he incised the fauces *aequalis sive par*, a phrase that presumably means 'symmetrically', and performed tracheotomy.[71] Soranus disapproves of such local incisions,[72] though he has been known to scarify the tongue in synanche.[73]

Caelius recommends venesection only when the disease is in remission,[74] but Asclepiades, in spite of his opinion quoted by Celsus that venesection at the height of the attack was equivalent to murder,[75] is said by Caelius to have venesected at the height of the attack in tetanus, since the peccant corpuscles, in his opinion, could not be withdrawn at any other time.[76] Asclepiades also, like Galen, believed that venesection might be called for in some geographical regions but not in others. This is not so, according to Caelius; to the Methodists the region in which the patient lives is of no consequence for the treatment.[77] Nor is the duration of the illness, in itself, of importance; unlike some who let blood only in the first three days, Caelius does so at any time when the patient's strength permits.[78] The fasting that must follow venesection is no contraindication to letting blood, if the patient's strength will stand both.[79] The operation, however, is

---

[65] Caelius, *CD* iii.65–6.   [66] Caelius, *CD* iii.65.   [67] Caelius, *CD* iii.61.
[68] Caelius, *CD* v.23. Others, according to Caelius, use music in the treatment of sciatica.
[69] Caelius, *AD* ii.156–7.   [70] Caelius, *CD* i.140–1.   [71] Caelius, *AD* iii.35.
[72] Caelius, *AD* iii.37–9.   [73] Caelius, *AD* iii.22.   [74] Caelius, *AD* iii.94.
[75] Celsus iii.18.6.   [76] Caelius, *AD* iii.93.
[77] Caelius, *AD* ii.129–31.   [78] Caelius, *AD* iii.12–13.
[79] Caelius, *CD* i.84; cf. Galen, who venesected and then fed the patient (K xi, 179, 199, 205).

equivalent to murder if undertaken when the patient's strength is impaired, as it commonly is after the seventh or eighth day.[80]

Revulsive treatment of haemorrhage by venesection is also mentioned. According to Caelius, it was undertaken by Hippocrates, Diocles, Praxagoras, Asclepiades, and Themison.[81] It would not be appropriate when a patient was already dying from haemorrhage.[82] Soranus and Thessalus venesected to stop bleeding on the third day, since, says Caelius, any wound that does not heal by that time must of necessity become inflamed.[83] As already mentioned, Caelius says that Erasistratus did use venesection to stop haemorrhage.[84] But many of Soranus' sect condemn this practice, on the grounds that venesection is a purely relaxing treatment and hence always inappropriate in a condition of looseness. Thessalus used it on the third day because he believed that at that time stricture predominated. Others employ it at once in all cases of haemorrhage, especially when this is copious or comes from the chest or lung. They seek to deflect the flow of blood, says Caelius, and also to withdraw excessive blood; the remedy may be applied repeatedly. So Themison used venesection both to relax and to lessen the amount of blood, thus preventing inflammation. Others think that the function of bleeding is to drain blood from ruptured parts, so that they may unite more quickly. Asclepiades held that the aim of venesection was to lessen the movement of the blood and of respiration, since this aggravated the disease.[85]

If, says Caelius, as Erasistratus believes, anastomosis (opening of the normally closed ends) of veins, due to a plethos of blood, might lead to bleeding, it is proper to use venesection, since the slight damage it does to the patient's strength is readily repaired.[86] At the same time, venesection should not be used for all patients who bleed. It is harmful where there is no obvious inflammation, as it leads to weakness, loss of appetite, and delayed healing of wounds. The bleeding is not stopped but only divided, so that the patient bleeds to death from two outlets instead of one.[87]

In all the foregoing discussion there is no mention of the site, or side of the body, at which revulsive venesection should be performed.

[80] Caelius, *AD* i.87.   [81] Caelius, *CD* ii.184.   [82] Caelius, *AD* iii.206.
[83] Caelius, *CD* ii.171–2.
[84] Caelius, *CD* ii.183.
[85] Caelius, *CD* ii.183–6. These comments are valuable in that they mention the rationale for venesection, a rare thing among the ancient writers.
[86] Caelius, *CD* ii.190. The Latin reads *osculatio venarum ex redundantia materiae*. Caelius does not say here that venesection was Erasistratus' treatment.
[87] Caelius, *CD* ii.190–1.

Caelius gives an interesting account of the views of various authorities, including Erasistratus, on the causation of haemorrhage.[88]

Lastly, Caelius recommends venesection as a treatment for severe toothache.[89] He also puts drugs into the ear opposite to the side affected, though others use the nostril on the affected side for this purpose. He does not, however, mention the side on which the venesection is performed.[90]

It seems clear enough from these extracts that there was little agreement on the part of other authorities, either with Galen or with one another, on the point in question. Why, then, did Galen believe in revulsive bloodletting from the affected side of the body? It would seem to a modern observer that his own dissections ought to have convinced him that there was no anatomical basis for his belief; the practice was by no means universal among his contemporaries and predecessors, and the Hippocratic writings exercised no infallible authority. Galen is so rational elsewhere, even if his premises are wrong, that it is strange to find him behaving, as it would seem, so very irrationally here. There are, of course, many practitioners today, even in the orthodox profession, who base their treatment on theories that no informed, intelligent and unprejudiced observer could possibly hold; one expects better, however, of a man of Galen's ability. It appears to a modern that Galen's anatomy is incompatible with his therapeutic methods; but Galen evidently saw the matter in a totally different light, since he appeals to anatomical demonstrations to justify his practice. In his work *On Tremor*, speaking of the maidservant of Stymargos[91] and Hippocrates' reasons for bleeding from the legs, he says:

That it is necessary to use phlebotomy when there is a plethos of blood is, I think, clear to everyone, for the blood is contained in the veins; but you would not be able to follow the argument that in disorders of the uterus the incision must be made in the region of the ankles or in the ham, unless I were first to demonstrate to you, by dissection, the connections of the veins. For a particular vein communicates with a particular part of the body, and one must always make the evacuation through connecting veins. If you were to incise veins that do not communicate at all with the affected part, you would not heal the affected part, and you would always do damage to the healthy one.[92]

At the end of his work *On the Natural Faculties*, Galen compares blood vessels to the irrigation system of a garden:

[88] Caelius, CD II.121–8.   [89] Caelius, CD II.74.   [90] Caelius, CD II.81–2.
[91] See above, p. 113, n. 10.   [92] K VII, 604.

You may learn this most clearly from irrigation furrows in gardens. For from these furrows some moisture is distributed to all the parts lying alongside and nearby, but it cannot reach to the more distant parts, and hence the gardeners have to arrange the flow of water to each part of the garden by cutting many small furrows leading off the big one, and they make the spaces between these small furrows of such a size as they think will best allow them to benefit by drawing from the moisture that flows to them from every side. It is the same in the bodies of animals. Numerous conduits distributed through all the limbs bring them blood just as an irrigation system distributes water in gardens.[93]

To reconstruct Galen's ideas we may therefore liken the body to a large level garden, watered by a spring in the middle; this corresponds to the new blood that is forming in the first veins in the region of the liver. From here, irrigation furrows lead in various directions. The diagram below shows only the principal furrows; they must be

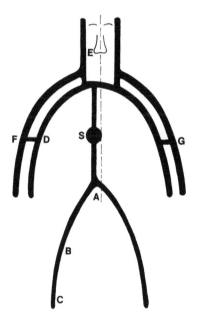

imagined as giving rise to many smaller ones, which in their turn do the same, so that no part of the garden is without some furrows close at hand. The ultimate subdivisions of the furrows end blindly, and the water in them soaks into the ground to nourish the plants; as it soaks in at the periphery it is constantly being replaced from the spring at the centre, so as to keep the furrows full. There is no circulation or rapid movement of water at all, only a slow seeping from the centre to the

[93] K II, 210–11. Elsewhere (K II, 23) Galen compares the veins to roads.

periphery to make up the loss there. It is not possible to stretch the analogy to account satisfactorily for Galen's two kinds of plethos, since for dynamic plethos to exist we would have to suppose an eliminative faculty in either the plants or the soil; plethos by filling, however, might perhaps be compared to a waterlogged state of the soil in a part of the garden, with the furrows overflowing and tending to disintegrate. Any kind of plethos requires evacuation before the plants suffer from an excess of water; this is achieved by making a breach in the wall and allowing the water to escape, presumably into a low-lying region which might be imagined as lying adjacent to the garden. Not all the furrows are accessible to such treatment; one cannot, for example, let blood from the vena cava.

Now suppose a woman whose menstrual catharsis has been suppressed. We wish her to bleed from the uterus at point A in the diagram, near the bifurcation of the inferior vena cava. It is obvious, on Galen's model, that if we open a vein in her leg or foot, at B or C, we shall draw more blood from the spring into the lower part of the vena cava, and this may cause the flow to appear. If, however, we open a vein in the arm, say at D, blood will be drawn in the opposite direction, into the upper part of the body and away from the lower part, and this will make her less likely to bleed from the uterus; it can in fact be used, he thinks, to reduce the menstrual flow if it is excessive. When a plethos is just beginning, therefore, the aim is to draw the blood away to a point as far as possible from the affected part. But once a plethos is well established there is no point in such a practice; when the soil in a particular spot is waterlogged, we must operate as close to the affected part as possible. Hence Galen's belief that incipient inflammations must be treated by revulsing or leading off (German *Ableitung*) of the blood in another direction, while established ones are to be evacuated as near as possible to the lesion.

A patient bleeding from the right nostril, at E, must according to Galen be revulsed on the same side of the body. The region at E is nourished by the vein that encircles the clavicle (modern external jugular) and if this vein could be opened the haemorrhage would be stopped by derivation. It was not Galen's practice, however, to open veins in the neck, and the accessible vein that was most directly connected with the one concerned was therefore used; this is the humeral (modern cephalic) in the right arm, at F. To use the humeral in the left arm would draw blood first from the parts most intimately connected with it, which are those of the left side of the face, and this would merely weaken the patient without having a prompt effect on the right side of the face at which treatment is directed. Galen was well aware that there were interconnections between all the veins, as there are between the furrows in the garden, but prompt results were desired; no gardener, after all, would open the furrow at G when the land at E needed draining.

It is not so easy to explain Galen's practice of bleeding from the right arm for disease of the liver, and from the left when the spleen is involved. He would probably say that the liver lies chiefly to the right of the midline, and the spleen entirely to the left of it; these organs have many small veins that nourish them, most or all of which are on the corresponding side of the body. To open the inner vein at the elbow (modern basilic) on the appropriate side would have a quicker effect in communicating more directly with all these small channels.

As far as we can determine from the extant literature, then, there is no evidence that there was in Galen's time a strong and orthodox body of opinion which held that blood ought to be let only from the affected side of the body. Galen's decided views on the subject appear to have been almost peculiar to himself. To the modern reader, who is aware of Galen's advanced anatomical knowledge, they seem at first sight quite irrational. Such a reader must remember, however, that while Galen's anatomy might be transferred almost unaltered into a modern textbook, the same cannot be said of his physiology. His ideas of the movement of the blood in the veins were quite unlike those that prevail today. Not only did his blood move in the opposite direction in the veins, but it moved very slowly. Once his revulsive practices are examined from his own point of view rather than that of a modern, it becomes clear that his advanced anatomy, far from contradicting them, in fact lends them support. It is true that it might be easier to justify them by appealing to one of the earlier anatomists, but they are still compatible with Galen's anatomy, as he himself obviously believed. The problem is not with Galen's anatomy, but with his physiology, and he can be understood by a modern only if he is considered in an out-of-date way. In the light of the knowledge of his time, his ideas on revulsion made sense.

In addition to his ideas about sites for revulsive venesection, however, Galen also believed, in common with many other practitioners of his day, in the efficacy of venesection as a general evacuant remedy. Today such treatment, except for a few special indications, is quite out of date. Was he wrong in this too?

CHAPTER 10

Galen's use of venesection as an evacuant: can it be justified? A medical digression

An aim of this work has been to examine, not only Galen's opinions on bloodletting, but also the reasons why he held them; it is therefore necessary to consider whether he could have been justified in believing what he did. Galen, like most other practitioners of his time, used phlebotomy as an evacuant remedy in a great variety of diseases; he also employed it as a revulsive in a way that would seem quite incompatible with his knowledge of anatomy, yet which can be shown to have been justified in the light of the knowledge of his time. Is there any scientific justification for his use of venesection as a general evacuant, taking into account that the conditions under which Galen practised were different from those now prevailing? The arguments to be put forward would not be accepted by all authorities today; it is nevertheless however possible for a professional haematologist, making use of discoveries in medicine in the last thirty years, to put up a case of sorts for Galen's use of venesection as an evacuant remedy. Any such retrospective evaluation must, of course, be highly speculative. Two separate arguments can be used; one concerns resistance to infection, while the other is rheological. Infection will be considered first.

Most physicians today, if asked whether there were advantages to the patient in being anaemic, would probably not be able to think of many. And although most would certainly agree that degenerative disease of the heart and arteries is less prevalent in the undernourished, the orthodox view is that impaired nutrition makes for greater susceptibility to infectious disease. This is the theme of a recent work by McKeown,[1] in which he argues that the notable rise in population since the Industrial Revolution has been due, not to advances in medicine, but to improvements in agriculture leading to better nutrition, with a consequent increased resistance to infection.

There is no doubt that there is much in this view. One of the

---

[1] T. McKeown, *The modern rise of population* (1976). He remarks (p. 157): 'Extensive experience in developing countries now leaves no doubt that malnourished populations have higher infection rates and are more likely to die when infected.'

reasons, however, why medical problems are so complex and unpredictable is that their causation is commonly anything but simple. What finally happens is always the resultant of a number of forces, some quite unknown and the majority incompletely understood, operating in different directions.[2] It should surprise no one, therefore, to discover that in some ways impaired nutrition might actually increase resistance to infection. It has, in fact, recently been argued that this is an evolutionary necessity, preventing on one hand the total extinction of the population when food is scarce, and on the other its unbridled increase in times of plenty.[3] It is not, however, necessary to consult the *Lancet* for 1977 to find this view expressed; the author of *Nature of Man* in the Hippocratic corpus, twenty-three centuries earlier, had observed that the proper course to take during epidemics was to keep the body as thin and weak as possible.[4] There is also the statement, which appears several times in the Corpus, that the condition of the trained athlete is unnatural and dangerous.[5] Turning to the special case of iron-deficiency anaemia, there is evidence that cell-mediated immune responses are depressed in this condition,[6] so that susceptibility to certain infections, particularly with viruses, might be expected to be increased; but there is some evidence that points in the other direction. In the nineteenth century Trousseau, a most experienced clinician, could write as follows:

When a very young physician, I was called to see the wife of an architect, suffering from neuralgia, a pale woman, presenting every appearance of chlorosis; I prescribed large doses of a preparation of iron ... In less than a fortnight there was a complete change; the young woman acquired a ravenous appetite and an unwonted vivacity: but her gratitude and my delight did not last long ... A short cough supervened, and in less than a month from the commencement of the treatment, there appeared signs of phthisis which nothing could impede,

and, concerning another patient,

a girl of fifteen, who after a mild attack of dothinenteria fell into a state of anaemia and prostration, which I considered chlorosis. I administered ferruginous remedies, which rapidly restored her to florid health; and although there

[2] Erasistratus denied causation in medicine altogether, because a particular alleged cause did not invariably lead to the particular effect expected. Celsus (Prooem. 54, 58–61) takes him to task for this. Erasistratus was like those today who say that smoking cannot be a cause of lung cancer, because some person who smoked did not suffer from it.

[3] M. J. Murray and A. B. Murray, *Lancet* 1 (1977) 123–5. See also G. V. Mann, 'Food intake and resistance to disease', *Lancet* 1 (1980) 1238–9.

[4] L 6, 56.

[5] E.g. L 9, 110; L 4, 458–60; L 5, 670. See also Plato, *Republic* III, 404a; Celsus 1.1.1–3; Caelius, *AD* I.113 (quoting Asclepiades).

[6] D. H. M Joynson, A. Jacobs, D. M. Walker and A. E. Dolby, *Lancet* 2 (1972) 1058–9.

was nothing in the family history to lead me to fear the coming calamity, she was simultaneously seized with haemoptysis and menorrhagia, and died two months afterwards with symptoms of phthisis, which had advanced with giant strides. I do not blame the iron for having caused this calamity; but I do blame myself for having cured the anaemia, a condition, perhaps, favourable to the maintenance of the tuberculous affection in a latent state.[7]

Trousseau wrote that very few physicians shared his views, but that his conviction of their truth increased daily. Had he been alive a hundred years later he might have seen them confirmed in the Ogaden desert, where famines are prevalent. Few of the inhabitants, while in a state of starvation, showed overt signs of infection with tuberculosis, malaria or brucellosis; but as soon as they were given a good diet in specially established relief camps, previously latent infections were immediately lighted up.[8] Similar observations have been made by other authors on human subjects[9] and on domestic animals.[10]

Since, in vertebrates, much of the iron in the body is in the haemoglobin, repeated loss of blood leads to an iron-deficiency anaemia. Not only men and animals, but bacteria and indeed all living cells require iron to sustain life and growth, and when bacteria invade the body they must get their iron from it if they are to multiply and bring about disease. In the last thirty years much has been learned about the competition for iron that takes place between the invaders and the body of the host. In 1946 Schade and Caroline described a protein in the blood plasma, transferrin or siderophilin, which has the ability to form a complex with iron that has been absorbed into the blood from the gut.[11] Because of this binding ability of transferrin, iron does not normally exist free (i.e. unbound to transferrin) in the plasma in any appreciable quantity. Estimations of serum (or plasma) iron measure the transferrin-bound iron in the liquid component of the blood; this is quite independent of the iron in haemoglobin molecules inside the red corpuscles. Because the transferrin in the plasma holds the iron so tightly, normal human plasma is not a good medium for the growth of many bacteria unless additional iron is added. Some bacteria, however, have developed their own compounds for binding iron; the tubercle bacillus, for instance, has one called mycobactin, which is effective enough to compete for iron with the transferrin in the host's plasma. In man, the transferrin is usually present in the

---

[7] A. Trousseau, *Lectures on clinical medicine*, vol. v (1872), tr. Sir John Cormack, p. 97.
[8] M. J. Murray, A. B. Murray, M. B. Murray and C. J. Murray, *Lancet* 1 (1976) 1283–5.
[9] H. McFarlane et al., *Brit. Med. J.* 4 (1970) 268–70.
[10] See the discussion in *Proc. Roy. Soc. Med.* 30 (1937) 1039ff.; particularly p. 1049.
[11] A. L. Schade and L. Caroline, *Science* 104 (1946) 340–2.

plasma in greater quantities than are necessary to bind the amounts of iron usually being transported; the percentage saturation of the transferrin is normally only about 30, so that unbound iron does not appear in the blood in any ordinary circumstances. At such relatively low levels of transferrin saturation the binding is extremely tight, so that unless invading bacteria have exceptionally active chelating agents of their own they will be unable to get any iron away from the host's transferrin, and consequently they will be unable to multiply in his body fluids. As the transferrin saturation increases, however, it becomes easier to induce it to part with some of its iron, and when it is fully saturated, iron can exist unbound in the plasma and bacterial growth is greatly enhanced.[12]

There is no doubt that these phenomena occur in the test tube; what happens in the body, however, may not be so simple.[13] Certain organisms, such as pyogenic cocci and pneumococci, multiply, in the host, in body fluids rather than inside cells. These are the organisms that are particularly susceptible to attack by humoral antibody, that is, specific immunoglobulin in the plasma and other body fluids, and the degree of saturation of the transferrin in these fluids might well – although it has not been proved in man – have a non-specific effect on their multiplication in the body. Other organisms, however, such as the mycobacteria (the causative organism of tuberculosis is a myco-bacterium) and Gram-negative bacteria multiply inside cells, sheltered from the body fluids; what goes on in the blood plasma, therefore, may be largely irrelevant in a disease like tuberculosis, in which the organisms are intracellular, inside the macrophages. Humoral anti-body against the tubercle bacillus, indeed, appears to be of very little importance in the defence of the body against tuberculosis. Biozzi and his co-workers have bred two strains of mice, selected respectively for high and for low humoral antibody response to certain antigens, notably those on the surface of sheep red blood cells. A surprising finding is that mice selected for high humoral antibody response to this restricted group of antigens are high responders to a very large proportion of other, unrelated, antigens as well, while mice bred for low response to sheep red cells are also low responders to most other antigens. It might be thought that it would be gravely disadvantage-ous to the low responder not to be able to mount an impressive humoral response to many common antigens, but there is in fact no evidence that low responders are on the whole any less healthy than high responders, and they are in fact more resistant than the high

[12] E. D. Weinberg, *Science* 184 (1974) 952–6.
[13] M. W. Mellencamp, M. A. McCabe and I. Kochan, *Immunology* 43 (1981) 483–91.

responders are to infections like tuberculosis. This is because their cell-mediated immunity, reflected in macrophage function, is better than it is in the high antibody responders,[14] and in diseases like tuberculosis it is what goes on inside the cell, rather than in the body fluids, that is important. But iron is involved here too, since the invading organism, wherever it chooses to lodge, must obtain iron from the host if it is to multiply significantly. It appears that intracellular organisms derive their iron from the host's ferritin, one of the substances used by the body to store iron inside cells.[15] The minute amount of ferritin circulating in the blood plasma can be measured, and this measurement has been shown to give a good indication of the total non-haemoglobin iron stores of the body.[16] Hence the plasma ferritin level probably gives an indication of the quantity of storage ferritin in the cells of the reticulo-endothelial system.

There is some recent evidence that ferritin may be important also in virus infections. Hepatitis B or transfusion jaundice is due to a virus which may also persist for long periods in the plasma of otherwise healthy people, known as carriers. This predisposes them to the development of primary carcinoma of the liver. It has been shown that in patients on haemodialysis, followed over many years, a high plasma ferritin level before there was any serological evidence of hepatitis B infection increased the likelihood that the infection, if it subsequently occurred, would be persistent.[17] One of the strange features of the epidemiology of hepatitis B is that men are much more likely, in most populations, to become carriers than women are; now that the connection with iron stores has been recognised, it becomes clear that this is probably because they have larger stores of non-haem iron, reflected in higher plasma ferritin levels.

In examining the possible effects of venesection, therefore, we must consider not only the transferrin saturation, which reflects the availability of iron in the body fluids, but also the level of plasma ferritin, which indicates its availability within cells. In fact the two measurements are usually correlated, in that iron-deficiency anaemia is marked by a decline in both; the critical question, however, seems to be the timing with which such a decline occurs.

Quite apart from iron-deficiency anaemia resulting from loss of blood, plasma iron falls sharply at the onset of bacterial infections in normal subjects; this may be a protective mechanism which makes it

[14] G. Biozzi et al., *Curr. Top. Microbiol. Immunol.* 85 (1979) 31–98.
[15] Mellencamp et al.
[16] A. Jacobs, *Semin. Haemat.* 14 (1977) 89–114.
[17] E. D. Lustbader, H.-W. L. Hann and B. S. Blumberg, *Science* 220 (1983) 423–5.

Table I: *Serum ferritin levels in new blood donors from two
population groups*

| Population | Sex | Number | Serum ferritin (µg/l) | |
			Mean	Std. deviation
White	Male	96	93	65
	Female	100	36	27
Black (Zulu)	Male	99	223	275
	Female	100	32	41

more difficult for the invaders to find nourishment.[18] A paper by the
Murrays deals with the effects of iron deficiency, uncomplicated by
malnutrition, in Somali nomads.[19] These who were iron deficient
showed significantly fewer infections than those whose haemoglobin
and plasma iron levels were more normal. Iron-deficient subjects were
then divided into two groups, one of which was treated with iron and
the other with an ineffective tablet or placebo. There were three
clinical episodes of infection among the 66 subjects in the placebo
group, as against 46 in the 71 subjects receiving iron. The authors
conclude that iron deficiency probably plays a part in suppressing the
clinical manifestations of certain infections. The infections they
encountered were interesting: the commonest was malaria, with
numerous recurrences of tuberculosis, brucellosis, and bacterial infections of the skin and eyes, very much like the medical problems of the
Hippocratic physician. Malaria was unquestionably the greatest
plague of the Greeks and of the ancient world generally, as Jones
points out in his general introduction to the Loeb Hippocrates; he also
mentions tuberculosis as one of the diseases that appears most
frequently in the Corpus.[20] These remarks apply to Galen's practice
too. Bacterial infections such as synanche and peripneumonia were
common. Is it possible that the patients of Hippocrates and Galen
were also, like the Somali nomads, party to an ecological compromise
in which iron-deficiency anaemia, the result of deliberate bloodletting
and of beneficial evacuations such as the menses and bleeding piles,

---

[18] Weinberg.
[19] M. J. Murray, A. B. Murray, M. B. Murray and C. J. Murray, *Brit. Med. J.* 2 (1978)
1113–15. They suggest that iron deficiency in these nomads may be part of an
ecological compromise. It is debilitating but rarely fatal, and prevents the more
serious consequences of infections such as malaria, tuberculosis and brucellosis.
[20] Hippocrates, Loeb Classical Library, vol. I, pp. lvi–lvii. We need look no further than
the girl from Chios (see above, pp. 44–7) for a case of tuberculosis.

protected them against worse evils in the form of life-threatening infections?

At least one infectious disease which is still common today, namely tuberculosis, provides some support for this view. Normal women of reproductive age are deficient in iron stores by comparison with men, as Table I, for South African voluntary blood donors from two population groups with different dietary habits, clearly shows.[21] This is presumably because of the blood they lose, since ferritin levels are similar in the two sexes before puberty:

Table II: *Median values for plasma ferritin (μg/l) in subjects of various ages*[22]

Age	10	20	30	40	50	60	70
Female	20	22	24	30	49	82	97
Male	20	32	97	108	122	129	144

Now in recent times – though it is not at all certain that this was so in the past – there is in most populations a very remarkable difference in the incidence of death from tuberculosis between the sexes. To quote a contributor to a work published in 1957:

... we see that for pulmonary tuberculosis at any rate, when statistics were first compiled a hundred years ago, there were more female than male deaths, but that very soon the males began to predominate and have done so ever since to an increasing degree until in 1950 there were 9 922 male deaths, and 6 047 female [in England and Wales]. Thus 62% of the deaths were in males. This is a remarkable difference, and in those parts of the country where the mortality is lowest, there the difference is most marked and sometimes 70% of the deaths are in males. So marked is this tendency that we have come to regard it as the way tuberculosis behaves when it is waning. The same phenomenon may be seen in the white population of the United States; in 1947 there were about 35 000 deaths in white people and of these 67% were in males. The male rate per 100 000 was 36.3 and the female was 18. Non-white deaths numbered 13 281 and of these 56% were in males. The male rate was 100.6 and the female 76. The same difference, though varying in degree, may be noted in other countries of Western Europe and the Dominions, and the temptation to regard the phenomenon as a law arises. Why should there be such a difference? There have been numerous attempts to explain it...[23]

---

[21] Data from Natal Blood Transfusion Service, Durban.
[22] Adapted, by permission, from Fig. 4.7 (p. 98) in T. H. Bothwell, R. W. Charlton, J. D. Cook and C. A. Finch, *Iron metabolism in man* (1979).
[23] F. R. G. Heaf (ed.), *Symposium of tuberculosis* (1957) p. 72.

The phenomenon, however, is not universal; at the time when this account was written the male and female death rates from tuberculosis were very similar in Holland, and in Iceland female deaths were more numerous. Hence any argument from these data should not be pushed too far. Again, the difference in death rates between the sexes tilts in favour of the females only at the age of about thirty; the difference in iron stores, however, as Table II shows, is evident at a much earlier stage. It seems clear, therefore, that iron stores cannot be the only factor responsible for the marked difference in incidence between the sexes. They may well, however, be one of the factors contributing to it.

In considering whether some such mechanism might have made it advantageous for the ancient physicians to use bloodletting, we must remember that the remedies at their disposal were very different from those in common use today. The first specifics, namely mercury for syphilis and quinine for malaria, were introduced only in Renaissance times, while sulphonamides and antibiotics for bacterial infections appeared only within living memory. It is true that venesection for the treatment of the acute fevers had virtually been abandoned before these last remedies became available, but this is not to say that, in the very different circumstances prevailing in antiquity, bloodletting was not of value. If, by its use, the ancient physician could prevent an infection which, once established, he was powerless to cure, he was justified in employing it.

Before we may assume that this was so, however, it is necessary to consider what the effects on transferrin saturation and iron stores might have been when patients in antiquity were subjected to Galen's system of venesection. This is, of course, highly conjectural; it must depend, not only on the amount of blood removed and on the frequency of venesections, but also on the iron content of ancient diets. This is of crucial importance because the iron stores of the body depend on it. A normal adult has about four grams of iron, about half of which is in the haemoglobin and the other half in the iron stores, principally in the liver. It has recently become possible to estimate these stores in a simple way, by determining plasma ferritin; one microgram of ferritin per litre corresponds, in normal subjects, to about 8 mg of iron in storage.[24] Iron is lost from the body in the faeces and sweat, and also, of course, in any bleeding that may occur; women of reproductive age therefore lose more iron than men do. It is taken into the body in food and drink, but not by any means all of the iron in the diet is absorbed. To some extent at least absorption is regulated by

[24] Jacobs.

the body's requirements, so that it is greater in iron-deficiency anaemia, but even here only a limited amount is absorbed. Iron is less readily absorbed from vegetarian diets than from those containing meat. If the amount absorbed is equal to the amount being lost, the stores remain constant and the subject is in iron balance. If more is absorbed than is lost, the balance is positive and stores increase; this occurs dramatically in many middle-aged black men in South Africa because of the large amount of iron in the traditional diet, and particularly in sorghum beer which is taken in large quantities. If more is lost than is absorbed, the subject is in negative balance and the stores decline. As long as some iron remains in the stores, loss of blood does not lead to a dramatic fall in plasma iron or transferrin saturation, though there is some effect on them; when the stores are exhausted, however, plasma iron and transferrin saturation fall notably, and the haemoglobin level declines as well, with signs of iron-deficiency anaemia in the peripheral blood.[25] The effects of bleeding, therefore, depend not only on the amount of blood lost and the frequency of bleedings, but also on the iron stores; and these, in turn, depend on the amount of iron in the diet. The effects of bleeding will be considered first; information is fortunately available from blood donors.

A single donation of whole blood, say 400 ml, removes about 200 mg of iron in the form of haemoglobin. Many donors give blood repeatedly at intervals which may be as short as two months, and may thus lose more than two litres of blood in the course of a year. It has been calculated that a daily loss of 6 to 8 ml of blood, say from bleeding haemorrhoids, may put a patient into negative iron balance even on a normal diet; this is the amount lost by a donor who gives regularly every two months. Laurell has published some figures on the effects of giving blood in Sweden just after the second world war.[26] Seventeen donors, most of whom had given only one previous donation several months earlier, were tested before and one week after donating 400 ml of blood. The mean serum iron was 117 µg/dl, and the mean transferrin saturation 37%, before the donations; a week later the means were 79 and 23 respectively. A group of 17 donors who had given repeated donations, totalling between 1.5 and 3 litres per donor in the preceding year, had a mean plasma iron of 95 µg/dl, and a mean transferrin saturation of 27%. These studies suggest that, at least in the dietary conditions then prevailing, the loss of even 400 ml of blood had some effect on plasma iron and transferrin saturation,

[25] Bothwell et al., pp. 44–5.
[26] C.-B. Laurell, *Acta Physiol. Scand.* 14, supp. 46 (1947), 82–90.

while the loss of two litres or thereabouts in the course of a year reduced both these levels considerably. Laurell also studied eleven patients with haematological signs of iron deficiency as a result of chronic bleeding from the gut or uterus; in these the mean haemoglobin level was about 8 g/dl, and plasma iron had a mean of 33 μg/dl and transferrin saturation 8%. These subjects would no doubt correspond to Trousseau's patients, and to some of those in antiquity who were enjoying beneficial evacuations from haemorrhoids or menorrhagia, which the doctors refrained from treating lest worse should befall them. Two observations of Galen's make this clear. He says that sometimes haemorrhoids bled so copiously as to kill the patient or to leave him hydropic or cachectic;[27] such losses would of course be treated. Sometimes, however, doctors deliberately provoked conditions characterised by bleeding, to get the advantage of beneficial evacuations in patients who were not already enjoying them.[28]

Further information can be obtained from the blood donors in Table I. Galen's moderate evacuation of three cotyles is the equivalent of two blood donations at once (800 ml); it removes about 400 mg of iron as haemoglobin. It should thus precipitate into iron-deficiency anaemia any person with a plasma ferritin of less than 50 μg/l, by exhausting the stores. Of the white donors in this table, 26% of the men and 81% of the women had ferritin levels below 50 μg/l. Thus the majority of the women, and an appreciable proportion of the men, would be rendered anaemic, or brought to the verge of anaemia, by just one of Galen's moderate evacuations, and few of either sex could withstand his more heroic ministrations, such as six cotyles at once, with haemoglobin levels intact.

The problem here, however, is not only whether a fall in serum iron or ferritin levels occurs, but exactly when this takes place. The decline in plasma iron that occurs at the onset of infection may begin during the incubation period, and is thus excellently adapted to serve as a protective mechanism for the host; a change delayed for some days, on the other hand, might be too late to have any beneficial effect. It would seem that loss of blood, at any rate to the extent of about 500 ml, an amount commonly given by a blood donor, might have this undesirable effect. Data were available for seven non-anaemic donors, all of whom had low plasma ferritins, varying from 5 to 27 μg/l; this is important since venesection might be expected to have little effect in the presence of substantial iron stores. On the first day after the venesection, plasma transferrin saturation had, in fact, increased rather than decreased in four of the seven subjects; on the second day

27 K xi, 307.   28 K xi, 170.

this effect was even more noticeable, with five increased, and on the third day the proportion was the same as on the first. Not until the seventh day after the venesection were almost all (six out of seven) of the subjects showing a decrease in transferrin saturation with respect to the levels before donation;[29] this is in agreement with Laurell's findings for the seventh day, already mentioned, but he mentions no studies earlier than that time. To venesect a patient with an already established infection, therefore – as the ancients were in the habit of doing – might well result, not in a lower, but in a higher transferrin saturation level during the crucial period of two or three days after the operation. We do not know, however, what the effect of bleeding is on patients whose serum iron has already fallen because of the onset of an infection; the subjects studied here were healthy donors who were not suffering from, or about to suffer from, any infective condition. For what the results are worth, however, they do not suggest that therapeutic venesection had any immediate beneficial effect by virtue of lowering plasma transferrin saturation. There is no doubt, however, that it reduces iron stores; this is a rapid process, and the effect on intracellular ferritin might be expected to be immediate. If therapeutic venesection works by denying iron to the invaders, it seems probable that we should look to the inside of the macrophage, rather than the body fluids, for the place where this effect takes place. And of course the objections above do not apply to prophylactic venesection, if sufficient to produce an iron-deficiency anaemia; here transferrin saturation would be reduced, and body iron stores exhausted, as a precautionary measure some time before infection took place at all.

The iron content of ancient diets is crucial to the argument. If most of Galen's patients consumed about the same amount of iron as Western man does today, his bloodletting would have more or less the effects mentioned. If, on the other hand, there was as much iron in their diets as there is in that of the average middle-aged tribal black man in South Africa, the effects of losing blood would be far less. André[30] has made a study of Roman diet, from which some idea of iron content can be obtained. The staple diet of cereals, vegetables and oil was clearly not particularly rich in iron; this must have been obtained chiefly from meat and from wine. There is, again, no evidence that the consumption of meat by the average man exceeded that of today; in the early centuries the Roman diet was in fact largely vegetarian, though more meat was eaten later. Unless we can discover some article of diet

29 Data from Natal Blood Transfusion Service.
30 J. André, *L'alimentation et la cuisine à Rome* (1961).

which both contained large amounts of iron and was taken in large quantities, like sorghum beer in South Africa, it will be unlikely that the average patient in Galen's time was far into positive iron balance. Some red wines today contain twice as much iron as traditional African beer,[31] although they are not usually drunk in such heroic quantities; nevertheless, some French wine drinkers become siderotic like some black Africans. It is possible, therefore, that the red wines of antiquity contained substantial amounts of iron; on the other hand, they were usually drunk diluted with water. The wine of poorest quality, from the later pressings of the material, might have contained more; this is particularly true of the worst kind, made by returning the exhausted skins to the press after they had been macerated in water. From such material the elder Cato prepared 'un horrible vin d'hiver' for his slaves, diluting 260 parts of this pressing with 1,500 parts of a mixture of fresh and sea water,[32] vinegar and heated wine. The ration for a slave engaged in the hardest labour was at most a litre a day,[33] which, allowing 100 mg of iron per litre in the original pressing, could scarcely, because of the dilution, have provided more than about 10 mg of iron, most of which would not have been absorbed. Slaves with lighter duties received only a quarter of this amount. Information about the diet of slaves in later and presumably more liberal times is lacking.

For the free man, consumption would depend on price. Under Diocletian, a century after Galen, half a litre of choice wine sold at the price of a kilogram of pork, while the same amount of *vin ordinaire* could be obtained for a quarter of this amount. André's conclusion is that the price of wine was never excessively high at any stage of Roman history, but was never so low that the poor could use it habitually. Athenaeus, who flourished at about the time of Galen's death, made the surprising observation that in his time women and slaves in Rome did not drink wine, while free men took it only after the age of thirty.[34] Galen, however, mentions the use of wine to bring on the menses,[35] and we have already seen that an earlier time of severer morals wine, if Cato's concoction can be so described, was not witheld from slaves. It therefore seems unlikely that Athenaeus was reporting the situation correctly, though it might well be that most women,

[31] Jacobs, pp. 98–9.
[32] Wine mixed with sea-water (*thalassomenos*) was used by Asclepiades, nicknamed the 'Winegiver', in treating the cardiac disease, a variety of circulatory collapse, since he believed it to flow rapidly and to reach all parts of the body (Caelius, *AD* II.228). He may have had in mind Euripides' line 'The sea cleanses all the ills of men', and seems to have anticipated the advertisements for a variety of beer which is said to refresh the parts that its competitors cannot reach.
[33] André, pp. 164–5.   [34] Ibid. pp. 170–1.   [35] K XI, 205.

through a combination of tradition and circumstances of life, drank less wine in Galen's time than their men did, thus unwittingly rendering their beneficial evacuations even more beneficial by taking a diet deficient in iron.

It is perhaps unlikely, therefore, that there was more iron in the diet of the average patient in Galen's time than there is in Western diets today, and many women were thus in negative iron balance; the same was probably true of a substantial proportion of men also. That this was so in Galen's time, if my thesis is correct, would appear from Galen's observation that women who had copious menstrual bleeding escaped many diseases, as did men who had bleeding haemorrhoids.[36] From an earlier period, we have also the observation of Aristotle that women were paler than men.[37]

A few years ago no one would have agreed that these evacuations might indeed have been beneficial; today it can at least be argued that they might have been. This observation by the ancients might very well have suggested to them the use of venesection, on the good Hippocratic grounds of assisting nature; when she was not evacuating enough blood by spontaneous haemorrhages, the physician ought to help her by venesecting. Even an empiricist might have argued in this way; those who accepted the humoral pathology had further theoretical grounds for letting blood.

The whole situation is complicated because there is no doubt that iron-deficiency anaemia, and undernutrition in general, have other effects that operate in the reverse direction, increasing the danger of infection by weakening the patient. Galen,[38] and the author of the *Appendix* to *Regimen in Acute Diseases*,[39] were well aware of the need to take the patient's strength into account before undertaking venesection. From Galen's statement, however, that all the empiricists used venesection, simply because experience had shown it to be valuable,[40] we may conclude that in the particular circumstances then prevailing, and when the patient's strength was carefully taken into account before undertaking the operation, the good effects of reducing the availability of iron to pathogenic organisms usually outweighed the bad effects of weakening the patient. That such good effects, in reducing the liability to infectious disease, may in fact occur – it cannot be claimed with certainty that they do – has only recently become known. It seems clear, however, that the balance was a delicate one; the advantages of using venesection did not so manifestly outweigh

---

[36] K xi, 165–6.   [37] *Generation of Animals* i, xix.
[38] For numerous references see above, p. 131, n. 89.
[39] L 2, 398.   [40] K xi, 163.

the disadvantages as to convince all physicians, and competent practitioners like Erasistratus could do without it and still make a living and a reputation. The majority, however, made use of it; it is possible that they were not entirely misguided.[41]

The rheological argument is probably less relevant to the circumstances of antiquity, and will therefore be dealt with in less detail. An editorial in the *Lancet*[42] in 1979 opened with the words: 'Arguably, the most important property of blood is that it should actually flow.' To oxygenate the tissues in every part of the body the blood must flow freely, through vessels, in the capillary bed, that are of very small calibre. The viscosity of the blood is thus very important. It depends in part on the concentration of certain proteins, such as fibrinogen, in the plasma, but principally on the proportion of its total volume taken up by the red corpuscles – the packed cell volume or PCV. The normal PCV is a little over 40%. The relationship between PCV and viscosity is not linear; at low PCV small changes in the cell mass have little effect on viscosity, but at PCVs in the region of 45% the effect may be considerable. Other things being equal, of course, the greater the PCV the greater the capacity of the blood to transport oxygen; but to do this it must flow freely to every part, like Asclepiades' *oinos thalassomenos*, and it cannot do this if its viscosity is too great. The remedy in such a case is to dilute it, as Asclepiades did his wine; bloodletting is still a recognised treatment for the condition of polycythaemia, in which the PCV is abnormally high. Such dilution can be achieved by venesection because the restoration of lost red cells is a relatively slow process, while the restitution of fluid is rapid; thus for some time after the bloodletting, PCV is reduced. It has been suggested that the best compromise between free flow and oxygen-carrying capacity, at least in the dog, is achieved at a PCV of about 30%,[43] which would be regarded as pathologically low by most physicians. The writer of the editorial suggests that perhaps natural selection in the remoter past has favoured individuals who could afford to lose a pint or two of blood, and this seems logical since trauma must surely have been a greater hazard for primitive man than degenerative arterial disease. In today's world, where the risks are different and blood lost can in any case be quickly and safely replaced, it may be that most people have too high a PCV. A large British survey has shown that there is a distinct increase in mortality, in women, at levels of PCV above 46%,

41 The argument that bloodletting might have protected against infection by denying iron to the invading organisms has been put forward by M. J. Kluger, *Natural History* 87 (1978) 78–83, and independently by myself, *S. Afr. Med. J.* 56 (1979) 149–54.
42 *Lancet* 2 (1979) 184–5.
43 C. J. P. Yates, V. Andrews, A. Berent and J. A. Dormandy, *Lancet* 2 (1979) 166–8.

due largely to cardiovascular disease.[44] (Men were not included in this survey.) In another study, some patients with peripheral arterial disease, resulting in intermittent claudication, were benefited by having 500 ml of blood removed once a week for three weeks, lowering the PCV to 35% or less.[45] Amputations in diabetics with peripheral vascular disease healed well in another survey when the patients were relatively anaemic (haemoglobin less than 12 g/dl) but did not heal at all when it exceeded 13 g/dl.[46]

These findings, it is true, apply to patients with arterial disease. We do not know how important the mechanism is in normal subjects, but it is clear that it is possible to argue, on rheological grounds, that some degree of anaemia might not be altogether a bad thing. Ancient medicine was far more concerned with infection than with degenerative disease, however, and the relevance, if any, of the rheological argument to Galen's practice therefore remains to be established.

[44] P. C. Elwood, I. T. Benjamin, W. E. Waters and P. M. Sweetnam, *Lancet* 1 (1974) 891–4.
[45] Yates et al.   [46] M. J. Bailey et al., *Lancet* 2 (1979) 168–70.

CHAPTER 11

Conclusion

In the foregoing chapters Galen's opinions on venesection have been collected from his surviving works and compared with the views of the Hippocratic writers and of some of his other predecessors and contemporaries. What has not been resolved, and probably cannot be certainly decided at all, is the origin of Galen's opinions. Although he has a profound respect for Hippocrates, his opinions on venesection are Hippocratic only in the sense that they are those of a fictitious Hippocrates whom Galen has constructed for himself. Although the seeds of his ideas are to be found in the Corpus, they have grown by the time of Galen into something far bigger and more organised than is found in the Hippocratic writings. It is not clear where and when this growth took place. Although Celsus, like Galen, makes more extensive use of venesection than the writers of the Corpus do, his practice is in many ways quite different from Galen's, and the same can be said of Aretaeus, Antyllus and Soranus. What, then, was the origin of Galen's peculiar methods and beliefs? They are not truly Hippocratic, and a study of a few surviving sources between the writers of the Corpus and Galen suggests that they were far from universal among practitioners of ability and reputation. Where, then, did they come from, and why did he hold them so tenaciously?

This question might best be answered with another: Why did Galen succeed in his practice? A study of his three works on venesection can show not only what his opinions on the use of the remedy were, but a good deal concerning his personality and the conditions of medical practice among the upper classes in the time of the Antonines. Galen first came to prominence in Rome because of his public meetings and demonstrations, in which he had no hesitation in violently attacking his medical opponents, and Teuthras wished to have a record of the meeting with Martialius so that he might quote Galen's criticisms of him when visiting his own patients.[1] Clearly the modern rule of medical etiquette that forbids a doctor to speak disparagingly of a colleague had not even been thought of in Galen's time; he made his

[1] K xix, 14.

reputation by doing exactly that. He makes a revealing remark in his account of the meeting with Martialius in the tract *On His Own Books*. 'From that time on I determined not to teach publicly or to give demonstrations any longer, having succeeded in my practice beyond my hopes.'[2] This makes it clear that his aim in holding meetings was not simply to enjoy philosophical discussion, but to get patients; and that he quickly got them, despite the brashness of his personality, shows how hard he worked at it. The competition was severe, for Galen could not have been alone in employing such methods. In such a struggle only a man with very strong and well-defined individual views would have any chance of success, since it would have been impossible for him to attack and condemn his opponents if his own views and methods were the same as theirs. Galen, unlike the majority who adhered to a sect or school, proclaimed himself to be above all sects, maintaining that those who followed a particular authority in everything were slaves, even if that authority was Hippocrates.[3] This enabled him to attack all the sects, no doubt putting him at a considerable advantage.

It must not be supposed, however, that Galen's system was erected with this aim in view. He was unquestionably a man of great intelligence and ability, who could see the deficiencies as well as the good points of the various doctrines in the Corpus, on a selection of which – if on any single foundation – he constructed his system, which was supported by the infallible opinions of the Hippocrates he had invented.[4] Like all systems, it was imperfect, and many of its contradictions must have been clear to Galen himself; but no one in antiquity had anything better, and most of his competitors, lacking Galen's intellect, must perforce have had to accept their systems ready-made from one of the sects. Once Galen had put his system together, however, it turned out to suit his combative and boastful personality very well, and to be excellently adapted to succeed in the rat-race of medical practice in Rome.[5] It is very probable, therefore, that Galen's decided and individual views on venesection, as on other subjects,

---

[2] K xix, 15.   [3] K xix, 13.

[4] Smith (1979, p. 64) observes: 'Unlike the modern medical student, Galen had to choose the philosophical basis of his science from diverse competing theories. He made and refined his choice gradually and not without influence from his teachers.' This is certainly so, but Galen was an exceptional man; I would think it doubtful that the average medical student in his time exercised much more choice in such matters than the one of today does.

[5] For the competitive society of Rome and Galen's personality, see *Prognosis to Epigenes*, K xiv, 599–673, now available in a critical edition, with English translation, by V. Nutton; J. Kollesch, 'Galen und seine ärztlichen Kollegen', *Altertum* 11 (1965) 47–53; Smith (1979), p. 96; Nutton (1972).

were unique to him. Given Galen's methods of attacking his colleagues to provide publicity for himself, it was necessary to be unique to succeed; and he succeeded. This might partly explain why he held some of his more unlikely opinions, such as those concerning haemorrhages and revulsion on the affected side, so strongly to the end of his days; he had built his reputation on them, and they had not failed him.

If this is true, then Galen's methods of publicity, objectionable as they were, were deliberately used. This distresses Ilberg: 'The endless venomous abuse of the hapless opponent exceeds all limits; through it Galen does most harm to himself; it is clear that he was basically a low character.' Galen would surely not have agreed that these methods did him any harm; they brought him, after all, to the bedside of the emperor. Ilberg describes him elegantly, though perhaps with some exaggeration, as 'zänkischer, eigensinniger, tückischer Klopffechter, der mit schäumendem Munde den Gegner anfällt', maintaining that his fury did not in the least abate with advancing years.[6] The three works on venesection, considered in isolation, would suggest that it did, but recantations from Galen, such as he makes in the second work, are distinctly uncommon, and perhaps the circumstances were unusual. The question arises, however, to what extent such conduct was necessary if one was to succeed in practice in Rome at the time. Had Galen been of the moral stature of a Socrates, or even of the doubtless imaginary Hippocrates whom he portrays as the ideal physician,[7] the solution would have been obvious; he would not have practised in Rome. One may wonder, however, to what extent Galen realised that he was, in Ilberg's words, 'ein niedriger Charakter', or whether indeed, by the standards of the time, he was particularly low at all. He writes of his ideal physician, whom all doctors should strive to emulate, without any suggestion that he knows that he himself falls short of the ideal. The good physician must despise possessions, 'for it is impossible', he says, 'at the same time to engage in money-making, and to practise so great an Art; it is necessary to despise one of them, if you are to press on with all speed towards the other.'[8] Although I have suggested that Galen, in the passage just quoted, has the saying of Christ recorded in Matt. 6.24 or Luke 16.13 in mind,[9] there is, as far as I

[6] 'A quarrelsome, self-willed, spiteful brawler, who goes for his adversary foaming at the mouth' (Ilberg IV, 617).

[7] K I, 53–63.   [8] K I, 57.

[9] Brain (1977). The Greek is as follows: Matt. 6.24 (Luke is virtually identical): οὐδεὶς δύναται δυσὶ κυρίοις δουλεύειν· ἢ γὰρ τὸν ἕνα μισήσει καὶ τὸν ἕτερον ἀγαπήσει, ἢ ἑνὸς ἀνθέξεται καὶ τοῦ ἑτέρου καταφρονήσει· οὐ δύνασθε Θεῷ δουλεύειν καὶ μαμμωνᾷ.

Galen: οὐ γὰρ δὴ δυνατὸν ἅμα χρηματίζεσθαί τε, καὶ οὕτω μεγάλην ἐπασκεῖν τέχνην, ἀλλ' ἀνάγκη καταφρονῆσαι θατέρου τὸν ἐπὶ θάτερον ὁρμήσαντα σφοδρότερον.

know, no evidence that he even knew of the Christian doctrine that good works are valueless if the attitude of mind of the doer is wrong, or that it is a sin to speak uncharitably of others. If asked about his ideal he would perhaps have replied that he practised in Rome because he had a mission to educate, not to make money, and his enormous literary output would certainly confirm this. Galen frequently mentions undesirable traits in others which are far more evident to the reader in Galen himself, but this does not occur to him. Teuthras was a man of very frank disposition;[10] Galen was worse still, and the Erasistratean physicians must have found them an insufferable pair. Martialius, an old man, was somewhat spiteful and contentious;[11] if he refrained from replying 'tu quoque!' he was also a man of considerable self-control. 'The same man', says Ilberg of Galen, 'who treats his contemporaries so slanderously, complains about the *kakoetheia* of his colleagues!'[12]

It seems possible, therefore, that Galen was genuinely quite unaware of his own imperfections of character; his actions, though deliberate, were not wrong in his eyes. That he undertook his immense labours principally for his own glorification is probably true, but the motive is not unknown today, and among the Greeks of antiquity it was both more common and much more respectable. Of his competence there can be no doubt; I am not so sure about his intellectual honesty. It is easy to admire him for many of his qualities, and to dislike him intensely for others; what is not easy is to feel any kinship for the man, as one sometimes can, in a flash of insight, for a writer like Homer or Virgil. This, however, is not the test of a good physician. Had I lived at the time, I should have had Galen for my medical attendant; one doctor cannot offer another a sincerer compliment than that. He did his best for his patients, and if he did his best for himself too, there was a precedent for that:

ἀρνύμενος ἥν τε ψυχὴν καὶ νόστον ἑταίρων.[13]

---

[10] K xi, 193. [11] K xix, 13. [12] Ilberg iv, 617.

[13] 'To preserve his own life and bring his companions home' (*Od.* i.5). The order of Odysseus' priorities is particularly significant.

GLOSSARY

NOTE: Archaic terms, and those whose meaning in antiquity was different from their present one, are marked with an asterisk.

anasarca: generalised dropsy.

anastomosis*: in antiquity, the opening of the normally closed blind end of a blood vessel; in modern terminology, a communication between two vessels.

aneurysm: a dilated part of an artery.

angina*: in antiquity, an acute inflammation of the neck and throat.

arteriotomy: bloodletting by opening an artery.

atonia, atony: lack of tone, flabbiness.

axilla: armpit.

cachexia: a state characterised by weakness and wasting.

cacochymia*: an excess of one of the three pathological humours: yellow bile, black bile, or phlegm.

canthus: the corner of the eye, where the eyelids meet.

cardiac orifice: the upper entrance of the stomach, where the oesophagus joins it.

chlorosis*: iron-deficiency anaemia with a greenish colour of the complexion; the green sickness.

choleric*: abounding in yellow bile.

cicatrise: to heal with the formation of a fibrous scar.

clavicle: the collar-bone.

collyrium*: an eye ointment.

coryza: common cold.

cotyle*: a Greek measure of capacity, about half a pint or 280 ml.

crasis*: the mixture of humours, or of qualities, in the constitution of an individual; temperament.

crude humour*: the end product of too little heat in digestion, so that instead of useful blood an undercooked, cold and watery humour is the result.

cubital: pertaining to the elbow.

cynanche*: an acute inflammation of the throat; more or less equivalent to *synanche*, although Galen distinguishes the terms in his more pettifogging moods.

derivation*: diversion of blood from an affected part to a nearby one.

diaphoretic: provoking sweating.

177

diaplasis*: the process in development by which the parts are moulded into their proper shape and form.

diathesis*: in Galen's system, any stable state of the body, whether normal or abnormal. In modern usage, a disposition or tendency to certain diseases.

dogmatist*: member of a sect which based its system on logic.

dothinenteria*: typhoid fever.

dyscrasia*: an abnormal or pathological crasis (q.v.).

dyspnoea: difficulty in breathing.

dysuria: pain or discomfort on passing urine.

elements*: the four elements are earth, water, air and fire; there is a fifth (aether) in the celestial bodies, and in the innate heat centred in the heart. The elements are the building materials of homoiomerous substances, but are so intimately mingled in them that no element is individually discernible.

emphysema: an abnormal accumulation of air, e.g. under the skin or in the tissues of the lung.

empiricist*: member of a sect which based its system on experience only.

empyema: accumulation of pus in the chest or other body cavity.

epaphairesis*: repeated removal (of blood).

epigastrium: the upper part of the abdomen, below the ribs; hypochondrium.

epiglottis: the structure covering the entrance to the larynx.

epistaxis: nose-bleeding.

erysipelas: an acute inflammation of the skin.

eucrasia*: a good or healthy crasis (q.v.).

fauces: the region of the throat where the tonsils are situated.

first veins*: the veins leading from the bowel to the liver in which, in Galen's system, the blood is supposed to be formed from nutriment absorbed from the bowel.

flux, fluxion*: a flow of humours to a part.

habitus: body type or physique.

haematemesis: vomiting of blood.

haemoptysis: spitting of blood.

haemorrhoid: a pile.

hectic*: (of fevers), continuous; not remitting.

herpes*: a spreading or creeping eruption of the skin.

homoiomerous*: uniform in texture; having no structure (to the naked eye).

humour*: one of the four elementary fluids of the body: blood, yellow bile, black bile, and phlegm. *See* quality.

hydrops: accumulation of fluid; dropsy.

hypochondrium: the upper part of the abdomen below the ribs; the epigastrium.

ileus: intestinal obstruction* or failure of movement of the intestines.

induration: hardness.

inosculation*: communication between arteries and veins; anastomosis (q.v.) in its modern sense.

ischium: a bone of the pelvis.

lochia: the discharge from the vagina for some days after childbirth.

malleolus: the bony lump on either side of the ankle.

marasmus: wasting.

melancholia*: a condition due to an excess of black bile.

menorrhagia: excessive loss in menstruation.

metastasis*: in Galen's system, the movement of a body of humours from one part to another.

occiput: the back of the head.

paremptosis*: in Erasistratus' system, the passing across of blood from the veins to the arteries.

pepsis*: digestion; the conversion of nutriment into blood.

peripneumonia*: an acute inflammatory condition of the lung.

peritoneum: the membrane lining the abdominal cavity.

perittoma*: (alternative spelling, *perissoma*): a residue of nutriment; material either of no use to the body, or in excess of its requirements.

phlebotomy: bloodletting by opening a vein.

phrenitis*: madness or delirium.

phthisis*: (= 'wasting'), a chronic disease of the lungs; probably usually tuberculosis.

plethos, plethora*: an excess of blood.

pleura: the membrane lining the cavity of the chest.

pleuritis, pleurisy: inflammation of the pleura.

pneuma*: air or breath.

pneumatist*: member of a sect regarding pneuma as the principle of life.

popliteal: of the region at the back of the knee.

pound*: the Roman pound (*libra*) was about 12 ounces or 350 g.

ptisan*: a kind of gruel.

quality*: the four Aristotelian qualities are the Hot, the Cold, the Damp and the Dry; they are associated with the four humours (blood hot and damp, yellow bile hot and dry, black bile cold and dry, phlegm cold and damp).

residue*: see perittoma.

revulsion*: diversion of blood from an affected part to a distant one.

rheology: the study of the flow of fluids.

rheumatic*: in antiquity, a condition marked by the flow or descent of a humour on any part.

rigor: shivering. (Not in the other modern sense of rigidity.)

satyriasis: excess of lust in males.

scirrhous: (of a tumour) hard and fibrous.

scotomatic*: characterised by 'blackouts'.

serous: having the nature of serum, a thin watery fluid.

sphacelus*: gangrene.

splenomegaly: enlargement of the spleen.

symptom*: a symptom, for Galen, is anything abnormal that happens to a patient. Its meaning is thus wider than the modern one, of something that the patient experiences – e.g. pain – although the doctor cannot observe it. If he can, it is a *sign* in modern terminology.

synanche*: *see* cynanche.

syndrome: a group of associated symptoms and signs.

temperament: *see* crasis.

tetany: a condition marked by cramps and contraction of muscles.

transpiration: passage of fluid and vapour through the skin.

varix: a distended or varicose vein.

vena cava: the principal vein of the body, entering the right auricle of the heart.

venesection: bloodletting by opening a vein.

WORKS CITED

Ackerknecht, E. H., 'Diathesis: the word and the concept in medical history', *Bull. Hist. Med.* 56 (1982) 317–25.

Allbutt, C., *Greek medicine in Rome*. London, 1921.

André, J., *L'alimentation et la cuisine à Rome*. Paris, 1961.

Anonymus Londinensis. *The medical writings of Anonymus Londinensis*, tr. W. H. S. Jones. Cambridge, 1947.

Aretaeus, ed. C. Hude. Berlin, 1958.

Aristotle
  Generation of Animals, tr. A. L. Peck. London & Cambridge, Mass. Loeb Classical Library, 1963.
  Historia Animalium, tr. A. L. Peck. London & Cambridge, Mass. Loeb Classical Library, 1965.
  On Respiration, tr. W. S. Hett. London & Cambridge, Mass. Loeb Classical Library, 1964.
  Pseudo-Aristotle, *On the Cosmos*, tr. D. J. Furley. London & Cambridge, Mass. Loeb Classical Library, 1965.

Bailey, M. J., Johnston, C. L. W., Yates, C. J. P., Somerville, P. G. and Dormandy, J. A., 'Preoperative haemoglobin as a predictor of outcome of diabetic amputations', *Lancet* 2 (1979) 168–70.

Bardong, K., 'Beiträge zur Hippokrates- und Galenforschung', *Nachr. Akad. Gött. Phil. Hist. Kl.* 7 (1942) 577–640.

Bauda, A., *Discours curieux contre l'abus des saignées* . . . Sedan n.d. (seventeenth century).

Bauer, J., *Geschichte der Aderlässe*. München, 1870.

Biozzi, G., Mouton, D., Sant'Anna, O. A., Passos, H. C., Gennari, M., Reis, M. H., Ferreira, V. C. A., Heumann, A. M., Bouthillier, Y., Ibanez, O. M., Stiffel, C. and Siqueira, M., 'Genetics of immune responsiveness to natural antigens in the mouse', *Curr. Top. Microbiol. Immunol.* 85 (1979) 31–98.

Bothwell, T. H., Charlton, R. W., Cook, J. D. and Finch, C. A., *Iron metabolism in man*. Oxford, 1979.

Brain, P., 'Galen on the ideal of the physician', *S. Afr. Med. J.* 52 (1977) 936–8.

Brain, P., 'In defence of ancient bloodletting', *ibid.* 56 (1979) 149–54.

Brock, A. J., *Greek medicine*. London, 1929.

Caelius Aurelianus, *On Acute Diseases and On Chronic Diseases*, ed. and tr. I. E. Drabkin. Chicago, 1950. (Cited as *AD* or *CD*, by book and section.)

Celsus, *De Medicina*, tr. W. G. Spencer. London & Cambridge, Mass. Loeb Classical Library, 1935.

Diller, H., 'Zur Hippokratesauffassung des Galen', *Hermes* 68 (1933) 167–81.
Dobson, J. F., 'Erasistratus', *Proc. Roy. Soc. Med.* pt. 3 (1927) 825–32.
Edelstein, L., *Ancient medicine: selected papers of Ludwig Edelstein*, ed. O. and C. L. Temkin. Baltimore, 1967.
Eichholz, D. E., 'Galen and his environment', *Greece & Rome* 20 (1951) 60–71.
Elwood, P. C., Benjamin, I. T., Waters, W. E. and Sweetnam, P. M., 'Mortality and anaemia in women', Lancet 1 (1974) 891–4.
Fraser, P. M., *Ptolemaic Alexandria*. 3 vols., Oxford, 1972.
Furley, D. J. and Wilkie, J. S., *Galen on respiration and the arteries*. Princeton, 1984.
Galen
    Claudii Galeni opera omnia, editionem curavit C. G. Kühn. 22 vols., Hildesheim, 1964 (reprint). (Cited as K by volume and page.)
    Galen on the Natural Faculties, tr. A. J. Brock. London & Cambridge, Mass. Loeb Classical Library, 1916.
    Galen on Prognosis, ed., tr. and comm. V. Nutton. Berlin, 1978.
    Galen on the Usefulness of the Parts of the Body, tr. M. T. May. 2 vols., Ithaca, 1968.
    Galen on the Doctrines of Hippocrates and Plato, ed., tr. and comm. P. de Lacy. 2 vols., Berlin, 1980.
Green, R. M., *A translation of Galen's Hygiene*. Springfield, 1951.
Goodfield, G. J., *The growth of scientific physiology*. London, 1960.
Graves, R. J., *Clinical lectures on the practice of medicine*. 2 vols., London, 1884.
Gray's Anatomy, descriptive and applied, ed. T. B. Johnston and J. Whillis, 28th ed., London, 1945.
Hammond, N. G. L. and Scullard, H. H., *The Oxford classical dictionary*, 2nd ed. Oxford, 1970.
Harris, C. R. S., *The heart and the vascular system in ancient Greek medicine*. Oxford, 1973.
Heaf, F. R. G. (ed.), *Symposium of tuberculosis*. London, 1957.
Hippocrates
    Oeuvres complètes d'Hippocrate, traduction nouvelle avec le texte grec en regard . . . par É. Littré. 10 vols. Amsterdam, 1962 (reprint). (Cited as L with volume and page.)
    Hippocrates, tr. W. H. S. Jones. 4 vols., London & Cambridge, Mass. Loeb Classical Library, 1923 and subsequently.
    Hippocrate, ed. and tr. R. Joly. Paris, 1972.
Ilberg, J. 'Ueber die Schriftstellerei des Klaudios Galenos', *Rh. Mus.* 44 (1889) 207–39 (i); 47 (1892) 489–514 (ii); 51 (1896) 165–96 (iii); 52 (1897) 591–623 (iv). (Cited by Roman figures as above, with page.)
Jacobs, A., 'Iron overload – clinical and pathological aspects', in *Iron excess: aberrations of iron and porphyrin metabolism*, i. Semin. Hemat. xiv (1977) 89–114.
Jaeger, W., *Diokles von Karystos: die griechische Medizin und die Schule des Aristoteles*. 2nd ed., Berlin, 1963.
Joynson, D. H. M., Jacobs, A., Walker, D. M. and Dolby, A. E., 'Defect of cell-mediated immunity in patients with iron-deficiency anaemia', *Lancet* 2 (1972), 1058–9.

Kluger, M. J., 'The history of bloodletting', *Natural History* 87 (1978) 78–83.

Kollesch, J., 'Galen und seine ärztlichen Kollegen', *Altertum* 11 (1965) 47–53.

Kotrc, R. F., 'Galen's On Phlebotomy against the Erasistrateans in Rome'. Unpublished PhD dissertation, University of Washington, 1970.

Kotrc, R. F., 'Critical notes on Galen's De venae sectione adversus Erasistrateos Romae degentes (K xi, 187–249)', *Class. Quart.* 23 (1973) 369–74.

Kotrc, R. F., 'A new fragment of Erasistratus' 'H ΤΩΝ 'ΥΓΙΕΙΝΩΝ ΠΡΑΓΜΑΤΕΙΑ', *Rh. Mus.* 120 (1977) 159–61.

Kudlien, F., 'A new testimony for Erasistratus?', *Clio Medica* 15 (1981) 137–42.

The Lancet, editorial 'Haemoglobin and the ischaemic foot', *Lancet* 2 (1979) 184–5.

Laurell, C.-B., 'Studies on the transportation and metabolism of iron in the body', *Acta Physiol. Scand.* 14, supp. 46 (1947) 1–129.

Liddell, H. G., Scott, R. and Jones, H. S., *A Greek–English lexicon*, 9th ed. Oxford, 1968. (Cited as LSJ.)

Lloyd, G. E. R., 'A note on Erasistratus of Ceos', *J. Hellen. Stud.* 95 (1975) 172–5.

Lonie, I. M., 'Erasistratus, the Erasistrateans, and Aristotle', *Bull. Hist. Med.* 38 (1964) 426–43.

Lonie, I. M., *The Hippocratic treatises 'On Generation', 'On the Nature of the Child', 'Diseases IV'*. Berlin, 1981.

Lustbader, E. D., Hann, H.-W. L. and Blumberg, B. S. 'Serum ferritin as a predictor of host response to hepatitis B virus infection', *Science* 220 (1983) 423–5.

Lytton, D. G. and Resuhr, L. M., 'Galen on abnormal swellings', *J. Hist. Med.* 33 (1978) 531–49.

McFarlane, H., Reddy, S., Adcock, K. J., Adeshina, H., Cooke, A. R. and Akene, J., 'Immunity, transferrin and survival in kwashiorkor', *Brit. Med. J.* 4 (1970) 268–70.

McKeown, T., *The modern rise of population*. London, 1976.

Mann, G. V., 'Food intake and resistance to disease', *Lancet* 1 (1980) 1238–9.

Marganne, M.-H., 'Sur l'origine hippocratique des concepts de révulsion et de dérivation', *L'Antiquité classique* 49 (1980) 115–30.

Mellencamp, M. W., McCabe, M. A. and Kochan, I., 'The growth-promoting effect of bacterial iron for serum-exposed bacteria', *Immunology* 43 (1981) 483–91.

Mewaldt, J., 'Galenos über echte und unechte Hippocratica', *Hermes* 44 (1905) 111–34.

Murray, M. J., Murray, A. B., Murray, M. B. and Murray, C. J., 'Somali food shelters in the Ogaden famine and their impact on health', *Lancet* 1 (1976) 1283–5.

Murray, M. J. and Murray, A. B. 'Starvation suppression and refeeding activation of infection: an ecological necessity?' *Lancet* 1 (1977) 123–5.

Murray, M. J., Murray, A. B., Murray, M. B. and Murray, C. J. 'The adverse effect of iron repletion in the course of certain infections', *Brit. Med. J.* 2 (1978) 1113–15.

Niebyl, P. H., 'Galen, van Helmont, and blood letting', in *Science, medicine and society in the Renaissance*, ed. A. G. Debus, vol. ii, 13–23, London, 1972.

Nutton, V., 'Galen and medical autobiography', *Proc. Camb. Philol. Soc.* 18 (1972) 50–62.

Nutton, V., 'The chronology of Galen's early career', *Class. Quart.* 23 (1973) 158–71.

Nutton, V., 'The seeds of disease: an explanation of contagion and infection from the Greeks to the Renaissance', *Med. Hist.* 27 (1983) 1–34.

Oribasius, *Oribasii collectionum medicarum reliquiae*, ed. J. Raeder. 5 vols., Leipzig, 1928.

Paulus Aegineta, The seven books of Paulus Aegineta, tr. F. Adams. 2 vols., London, 1847.

Peterson, D. W., 'Observations on the chronology of the Galenic corpus', *Bull. Hist. Med.* 51 (1977) 484–95.

Plato, *Republic*, ed. J. Adam. Cambridge, 1909.

Rawson, E., 'The life and death of Asclepiades of Bithynia', *Class. Quart.* 32 (1982) 358–70.

Royal Society of Medicine. Discussion on 'Nutrition and its effects on infectious disease', *Proc. Roy. Soc. Med.* 30 (1937) 1039–52.

Saunders, J. B. de C. M. and O'Malley, C. D. *Andreas Vesalius Bruxellensis: the bloodletting letter of 1539.* London, n.d.

Scarborough, J., 'Galen and the gladiators', *Episteme* 5 (1971) 98–111.

Schade, A. L. and Caroline, L. 'An iron-binding component in human blood plasma', *Science* 104 (1946) 340–2.

Sider, D. and McVaugh, M., 'Galen on tremor, palpitation, spasm and rigor', *Trans. Stud. Coll. Phys. Philad.* n.s. 6 (1979) 183–210.

Siegel, R. E., 'Galen's concept of bloodletting in relation to his ideas on the pulmonary and peripheral blood flow and blood formation', in *Science, medicine and society in the Renaissance*, ed. A. G. Debus, vol. I, 243–75. London, 1972.

Siegel, R. E., *Galen's system of physiology and medicine.* Basel, 1968.

Smith, W. D., *The Hippocratic tradition.* Ithaca, 1979.

Smith, W. D., 'Erasistratus's dietetic medicine', *Bull. Hist. Med.* 56 (1982) 398–409.

Steuer, R. O. and Saunders, J. B. de C. M., *Ancient Egyptian and Cnidian medicine.* Berkeley, 1959.

Trousseau, A., *Lectures on clinical medicine* ... tr. P. V. Bazire and others. 5 vols., London, 1868–72.

Waterton, C. *Essays on natural history.* London, 1871.

Weinberg, E. D. 'Iron and susceptibility to infectious disease', *Science* 184 (1974) 952–6.

Wilson, L. G., 'Erasistratus, Galen and the pneuma', *Bull. Hist. Med.* 33 (1959) 293–314.

Yates, C. J. P., Andrews, V., Berent, A. and Dormandy, J. A., 'Increase in leg blood-flow by normovolaemic haemodilution in intermittent claudication', *Lancet* 2 (1979) 166–8.

INDEX

NOTE: Where a book or paper has more than one author, only the first is indexed.

For EU product safety concerns, contact us at Calle de José Abascal, 56–1°,
28003 Madrid, Spain or eugpsr@cambridge.org.

www.ingramcontent.com/pod-product-compliance
Ingram Content Group UK Ltd.
Pitfield, Milton Keynes, MK11 3LW, UK
UKHW010046140625
459647UK00012BB/1641